To Improve Health and Health Care

Volume X

JB JOSSEY-BASS

Stephen L. Isaacs and
James R. Knickman, Editors

Foreword by Risa Lavizzo-Mourey

To Improve Health and Health Care

Volume X

The Robert Wood Johnson
Foundation Anthology

BICENTENNIAL
1807
WILEY
2007
BICENTENNIAL

John Wiley & Sons, Inc

—ᘺ— Table of Contents

Foreword: Of Hedgehogs and Flywheels   ix
Risa Lavizzo-Mourey

Editors' Introduction   xvii
Stephen L. Isaacs and James R. Knickman

Acknowledgements   xxv

Section One: A Ten-Year Retrospective   1

1   Health, Health Care, and the Robert Wood Johnson
Foundation: A Ten-Year Retrospective, 1996–2006   3
Stephen L. Isaacs, James R. Knickman, and David J. Morse

Section Two: Quality of Care   23

2   The Dartmouth Atlas of Health Care   25
Carolyn Newbergh

3   Improving Chronic Illness Care   49
Irene M. Wielawski

Section Three: Insurance Coverage   77

4   Increasing Health Insurance Coverage at the
Local Level: The Communities In Charge Program   79
Mary Nakashian

5   The Partnership for Long-Term Care: A Public-
Private Partnership to Finance Long-Term Care   105
Joseph Alper

Section Four: Services for Vulnerable Populations   125

6 **Supportive Housing**   127
   Lee Green

7 **SPARC—Sickness Prevention Achieved Through Regional
   Collaboration**   145
   Paul Brodeur

8 **The Southern Rural Access Program**   169
   Digby Diehl

Section Five: The Robert Wood Johnson Foundation   197

9 **The Robert Wood Johnson
   Foundation: 1974–2002**   199
   Joel R. Gardner

10 **Engaging Coalitions to Improve Health and
   Health Care**   221
   Laura C. Leviton and Elaine F. Cassidy

   Afterword   245
   Stephen Isaacs

   The Editors   247

   The Contributors   249

   Index   255

   Tables of Contents of Previous Volumes   267

—ɯ— Foreword: Of Hedgehogs and Flywheels

Risa Lavizzo-Mourey

With the publication of the tenth volume of the *Anthology* series, the Robert Wood Johnson Foundation has reached a milestone. In his foreword to the first volume, my predecessor Steven Schroeder wrote, "The chapters selected for this volume offer only a glimpse of the richness and diversity of our interests. A more complete picture will emerge with the publication of future volumes of the anthology over the coming years."[1] A decade later, the *Anthology* has published more than 100 chapters that do, indeed, offer a more complete picture of the ways in which the Foundation has worked to fulfill its mission of improving health and health care for all Americans.

Because the appearance of a tenth anniversary volume is significant, I felt it would be appropriate for me to provide a context for the book by examining how the Robert Wood Johnson Foundation, in carrying out its mission, strives to be not simply a good philanthropy but a great one. I do not use the word "great" lightly nor do I wish to be immodest in stating our aspiration so boldly. But all of us—board and staff alike—take our work seriously and are committed to making the Robert Wood Johnson Foundation as great as it can be.

In this regard, we have benefited from the work of former Stanford Business School professor Jim Collins, whose two books, *Built to Last*[2] and *Good to Great*,[3] analyzed the factors that distinguished great companies from merely good ones. Collins extended his analysis to the nonprofit world in a recent monograph, *Good to Great and the Social Sectors.*[4] His thesis can be summarized succinctly: Greatness is largely a matter of conscious choice and discipline—disciplined people, disciplined thought, and disciplined action.

Applying this to the Robert Wood Johnson Foundation leads us to take away four lessons.

First, defining greatness for a philanthropy is less clear cut than in business, but it is essential to agree on a definition.

While the Foundation uses "impact" as a shorthand term, Collins would say that greatness for nonprofits must encompass superior performance and lasting endurance, as well as a distinctive impact. In other words, the Robert Wood Johnson Foundation can claim to have had an impact when it causes or facilitates enduring change in an area that improves health care delivery or people's health and thus their quality of life.

Inevitably, we fall into the trap of enumerating specific programs or actions that have caused enduring improvements in health or health care. Yet research suggests that it is not single blockbuster programs that produce impact but rather the combination of disciplined people's thoughts and actions that create greatness over a sustained period of time. The key is to rigorously and routinely assemble the evidence—be it quantitative or qualitative—that allows one to assess performance, discipline, and momentum.

Second, in order to be great, we must apply the Hedgehog Concept.

The Hedgehog Concept derives from an ancient Greek poem attributed to Archilochus of Paros which loosely translated says, "The fox knows many things, but the hedgehog just one big thing." In other words, the fox is scattered, diffuse, distracted. In contrast, the hedgehog simplifies the complexities of the world into a single unifying principle that guides all of its activity. Focused, determined, relentless.

Great organizations are disciplined in thought and action as they define the intersection of these circles and stay focused on it. This has been our biggest challenge. The temptation in philanthropy is to take on many things because they will do some good. In looking at the three circles comprising the Hedgehog Concept, we know that we are passionate about helping Americans live healthier lives. We know, too, that we do well training leaders in health care, incubating innovative models to deliver needed services to vulnerable populations, creating the evidence and advocacy that can drive policy change, and identifying the important

Hedgehog Concept

What are you
deeply passionate
about?

What do you
do best?

What drives
your resource
engine?

areas that have the potential to transform the health of the people we serve. Our resource engine is not the generation of revenue but rather the combined power of our financial assets and the intellect of our staff and grantees, from which our good reputation derives. Mastering the Hedgehog Concept is more difficult than depicting it, but I think we are making progress.

Robert Wood Johnson Foundation Impact Framework

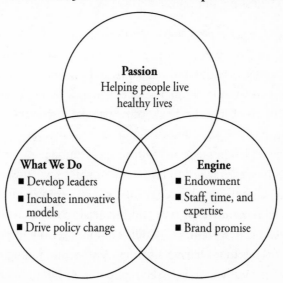

Passion
Helping people live
healthy lives

What We Do
- Develop leaders
- Incubate innovative models
- Drive policy change

Engine
- Endowment
- Staff, time, and expertise
- Brand promise

The Foundation's Impact Framework helps us stay focused on those things we do best. It groups our work into four different portfolios, sets goals, and assigns resources to each portfolio.

- By putting all the training and fellowship programs together in the Human Capital Portfolio and charging a group of staff members to think about workforce needs in health care, we stay focused on creating health care leaders—whether they be community health leaders, policy research leaders, or national leaders.

- The Vulnerable Populations Portfolio focuses on incubating innovative models to deliver care to the elderly, new immigrants, teenage mothers and their children, the chronically homeless, and others who are often marginalized or forgotten.

- The Targeted Portfolio takes a few areas such as quality, childhood obesity, public health infrastructure, and health care disparities, among others, and applies our ability to build an evidence base and to use it to advocate for the changes that will help Americans live healthier lives.

- Finally, the Pioneer Portfolio drives us toward continually incubating innovation.

Yet, even with a structured Impact Framework, we find it difficult to be disciplined and to say no to ideas and programs that are clearly worthwhile but do not fit within our portfolios and strategies.

A few words about the engine. More and more, we must fine-tune the firing of all of its cylinders—our financial assets, the dedication and expertise of the staff, and the Foundation's reputation. For many years, the Foundation made an effort to speak through our grantees. As I discussed in the foreword to last year's *Anthology,* we now talk about connecting, communicating, coordinating, and convening as deliberate strategic investments of staff and financial resources to speak *with* and *on behalf of* our grantees.[5] Collins emphasizes the importance of nonprofit organizations having a strong identity, and tuning the engine this way reciprocally enhances the reputation of our grantees and the Foundation.

Third, the Flywheel Concept describes the payoff.

Creating transformative impact—improving the health and health care of all Americans—suggests turning a giant flywheel. Remember the concept from Physics 101—a heavy wheel that is hard to turn until it gains momentum and then is almost unstoppable. The image of the flywheel I like best is that of the child-propelled merry-go-round. They were ubiquitous in the playgrounds of old. Do you remember the flywheels designed for us kids to grasp as we ran faster and faster until the merry-go-round's momentum swept us off our feet? Then we would jump on to the spinning disk, screaming as we reaped the joy of our collective effort. In Collins' words, "By focusing on your Hedgehog Concept, you build results. Those results, in turn, attract resources and commitment, which you use to build a strong organization. That strong organization then delivers even better results, which attracts greater resources and commitment, which builds a stronger organization, which enables even better results." People want to feel the excitement of being involved in something that just flat out works. When they begin to see tangible results—when they can feel the fly-

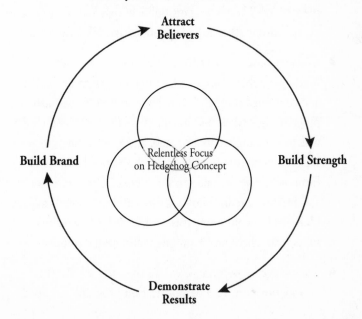

The Flywheel in the Social Sectors

wheel beginning to build speed—that's when more people line up to throw their shoulders against the wheel and push.

The Foundation's flywheel is gaining momentum. Consider, for example:

- *Significant changes in tobacco use and policy in the United States.* The Foundation has supported organizations working to affect the price of cigarettes, understand the impact of secondhand smoke, and establish clean indoor air policies. In December 2005, *USA Today* reported that 39 percent of Americans are covered by smoke-free laws or regulations (surpassing the Foundation's target of 35 percent by July 2006).

- *Care of HIV/AIDS patients.* In the 1980s, Foundation-funded hospital surveys documented the cost of care for HIV-positive patients. This led to Congressional testimony, then to funding of outpatient care for AIDS patients, and ultimately to funding for care of those with HIV-related illnesses. Foundation-funded demonstration programs provided the model for the Ryan White Act, the federal government's primary source of funds for care of people with AIDS.[6] At a 2004 *Time*/ABC News Summit on Obesity, Peter Jennings, the late ABC News anchor, publicly thanked the Foundation for the momentum it had generated in HIV/AIDS care.

- *Children's access to health care in schools.* The Foundation's funding of school-based health programs began in the 1980s and continued through 2005. These Foundation-funded programs helped expand the number of school-based clinics, which now number about 1,500, and enabled them to attract stable funding through Medicaid, the State Children's Health Insurance Program, and private sources.[7] The Center for Health and Health Care in Schools, located at the George Washington University, is continuing this work by providing technical support to school health programs around the country.

- *The emergency response system.* In the early 1970s, the Foundation funded a demonstration program that sped the development of the 911 emergency response system. Thereafter, President Gerald Ford signed legislation establishing a national emergency response system, based on the Foundation's work.[8]

- *Long-term care insurance.* In the 1980s, the Foundation began funding the development of public-private partnerships between insurance companies and state governments to make long-term care insurance more affordable and accessible. The policy research, demonstrations, and advocacy that began in four states recently paid off when the Deficit Reduction Act of 2005 authorized expansion of these partnerships to all fifty states.[9]

Even though the Foundation was often far from the sole actor in these examples, our leadership, funding, and persistence helped turn the flywheel of change. The best foundations have often been among the first pushing when the wheel is hardest to turn and is building momentum. As others join in, it picks up speed and energy. Many times, and I think appropriately, we curtail our financial commitment at that point.

In visiting dozens of impressive programs, I have often reflected on the momentum of the flywheel and how the Foundation can ensure continued momentum, even as our financial support declines. Many programs have been successful in developing innovative approaches to significant problems, achieving their goals, and attracting considerable attention. However, their potential for enduring impact has not been completely realized, and we will not understand their full effect for many years. We have to stay connected, enhance these programs by using our credibility on their behalf, and disseminate their results to teach others.

Fourth, and finally, an especially important lesson is reflected in the Foundation's third Guiding Principle that commits us to lifelong learning and continual improvement.

Collins says it this way, "No matter how much you have achieved, you are always merely good compared to what you can become. The moment you think of yourself as great, the slide to mediocrity will have already begun."

We are proud of improving the health of Americans through our work to develop leaders, nurture the field of health policy research, reduce the prevalence of tobacco use, and change the way people think of end-of-life care—to name the most frequently cited. We can be even better—even great—if we stay focused and disciplined about achieving tangible results and keeping all cylinders of our engine firing to turn the flywheel.

Princeton, New Jersey   Risa Lavizzo-Mourey
June, 2006   President and CEO
                              The Robert Wood Johnson Foundation

Notes

1. Schroeder, S. A. "Foreword." *To Improve Health and Health Care 1997: The Robert Wood Johnson Foundation Anthology.* San Francisco: Jossey-Bass, 1997.
2. Collins J. and Porras, J. *Built to Last: Successful Habits of Visionary Companies.* New York: Harper Collins, 1994.
3. Collins, J. *Good to Great: Why Some Companies Make the Leap . . . and Others Don't.* New York: Harper Collins, 2001.
4. Collins J. *Good to Great in the Social Sectors: A Monograph to Accompany Good to Great.* New York: Harper Collins, 2005.
5. Lavizzo-Mourey, R. "Foreword." *To Improve Health and Health Care, Vol. IX: The Robert Wood Johnson Foundation Anthology.* San Francisco: Jossey-Bass, 2006.
6. Bronner, E. "The Foundation and AIDS: Behind the Curve but Leading the Way." *To Improve Health and Health Care, Vol. V: The Robert Wood Johnson Foundation Anthology.* San Francisco: Jossey-Bass, 2002.
7. Lear, J. G., Isaacs, S. L., and Knickman, J. R. (eds.) *School Health Services and Programs.* San Francisco: Jossey-Bass, 2006.
8. Diehl, D. "The Emergency Medical Services Program." *To Improve Health and Health Care 2000: The Robert Wood Johnson Foundation Anthology.* San Francisco: Jossey-Bass, 1999.
9. See Chapter 5 of this volume.

~ᵐᵐ~ Editors' Introduction

Stephen L. Isaacs and James R. Knickman

Somewhat over a decade ago, Frank Karel, who was then the vice president for communications of the Robert Wood Johnson Foundation, and the two of us met in a small office at the Foundation and pondered how the Foundation might get reports and evaluations out of the bottom drawers of program officers' filing cabinets and into the hands of a broader public. We wanted to share knowledge of the Foundation's grantmaking and other activities with health policy makers and shapers; government health officials; staff members and trustees of foundations; health policy and program experts; people in the field working to improve health and health care; health policy researchers; members of the media; and the lay public interested in health or philanthropy.

From this and subsequent conversations involving many others at the Foundation emerged the idea of the *Robert Wood Johnson Foundation Anthology*. Our intention was, and is, primarily to give the broad array of readers mentioned above an understanding of what the Foundation has done to improve the health and health care of Americans, why it chose the paths that it did, and what lessons have been learned from its experience. Secondarily, we hope to demystify the Foundation by giving readers a glimpse of how decisions are made at the Foundation's headquarters in Princeton, New Jersey. We commission an array of writers—from professional journalists to program evaluators to Foundation staff members—and instruct them to write as honest and objective (and readable) an assessment of their topic as possible.

In its ten years, the *Anthology* has offered chapters on the range of ways in which the Foundation has addressed the nation's health and health care needs. Here is one way of illustrating the topics covered in the *Anthology* series:

Health Insurance Coverage and Health Care Policy

- National Access-to-Care Surveys (1997)
- The Foundation's Efforts to Cover the Uninsured (Vol. IX)
- Health Insurance for Children (2000)
- The Health Tracking Initiative (Vol. VI)
- Improving State Government Capacity in Health Reform (1997)
- Health Insurance at the Local Level: The Communities In Charge Program (Vol. X)
- The National Health Policy Forum (Vol. VII)

Access to Health Care Services and Cost Containment

- Safety-Net Programs (Vol. IX)
- The Medicaid Managed Care Program (Vol. IX)
- Academic Medical Centers (1998–1999)
- Managed Care (2001)
- Workers' Compensation (2001)
- Medical Malpractice (1997)
- Public Health: The Turning Point Program (Vol. VIII)
- Treating Tuberculosis (Vol. V)
- Dental Care (2001)
- Emergency Medical Services (2000)
- The Homeless Prenatal Program (Vol. VII)
- The Homeless Families Program (1997)
- Supportive Housing (Vol. X)
- The Southern Rural Access Program (Vol. X)

- Prevention Through Regional Collaboration: The SPARC Program (Vol. X)

- The Foundation's Efforts to Contain Health Care Costs (Vol. VII)

- Volunteer Physicians: The Reach Out Program (1997)

The Health Care Workforce

- The Health Care Workforce (1997)

- The Community Health Leadership Awards Program (Vol. VI)

- The Health Policy Fellowships Award Program (Vol. V)

- Building Capacity in the Social Sciences (Vol. VI)

- The Clinical Scholars Program (Vol. VII)

- Attracting Health Professionals to Underserved Areas: The Practice Sights Program (Vol. VI)

- Increasing Minorities in the Health Professions (Vol. VII)

- The Minority Medical Education Program (now the Summer Medical and Dental Education Program) (2000)

Children and Adolescents

- The Foundation's Children's Health Initiatives (2001)

- School-Based Health Care (2000)

- The Nurse Home Visitation Program (Vol. V)

- Immunization Registries: The All Kids Count Program (1997)

- Mental Health Services for Young People (1998–1999)

- Regional Perinatal Care Networks (2001)

- Preventing Injuries to Children (Vol. VII)

- The Chicago Program for Violence Prevention (Vol. VIII)

- Students Run LA (Vol. IX)

Nursing

- The Foundation's Nursing Initiatives (Vol. VIII)
- Strengthening Hospital Nursing (1998–1999)
- Nurse Practitioners and Physician Assistants (1998–1999)

Long-Term Care

- Long-Term Care Insurance: The Partnership for Long-Term Care (Vol. X)
- Consumer Choice in Long-Term Care (Vol. V)
- The Teaching Nursing Home Program (Vol. VII)
- Rural Hospitals and Long-Term Care: The Swing Bed Program (Vol. VI)
- Financing Affordable Long-Term Care Housing: The Coming Home Program (2000)
- Integrating Acute and Long-Term Care for the Elderly (2001)
- Service Credit Banking (Vol. V)

End-of-Life Care

- Research into End-of-Life Care: SUPPORT (1997)
- The Foundation's Programs to Improve Care toward the End-of-Life (Vol. VI)

Chronic Health Conditions

- Improving Chronic Illness Care (Vol. X)
- The Dartmouth Atlas of Health Care (Vol. X)
- Improving Health in an Aging Society (Vol. IX)
- Unmet Need in the Community: The Springfield Study (1997)
- Programs to Address Chronic Illness (1998–1999)
- Adult Day Centers (2000)

- The Program on Chronic Mental Illness (2000)
- AIDS (Vol. V)
- Community Volunteers: The Faith in Action Program (1998–1999)

Tobacco Control

- The Foundation's Tobacco-Control Strategy (Vol. VIII)
- Tobacco Policy Research (1998–1999)
- The National Spit Tobacco Program (1998–1999)
- The Sundance Conference and Its Aftermath (2000)
- Smoking Cessation (Vol. VI)
- The National Center for Tobacco-Free Kids (Vol. VI)
- The Smokeless States Program (Vol. VIII)
- Fighting Back (Vol. VII)
- Join Together and CADCA (Vol. VII)
- Free to Grow (Vol. IX)

Alcohol Use and Abuse

- Alcohol and Work: Results from a Corporate Drinking Study (1998–1999)
- Programs to Improve the Health of Native Americans (Vol. V)
- Recovery High School (Vol. V)
- Fighting Back and Healthy Nations in Gallup, New Mexico (Vol. VI)
- Reducing Underage Drinking (Vol. VIII)

Communications Initiatives

- The Foundation's Radio and Television Grants (1998–1999)
- Sound Partners for Community Health (2001)

- The Media and Health Systems Change (1997)

- The Covering Kids Communication Campaign (Vol. VI)

Inside the Robert Wood Johnson Foundation

- The Robert Wood Johnson Foundation's Early Years (Vol. VIII)

- The Robert Wood Johnson Foundation: 1974–2002 (Vol. X)

- An Interview with Steven Schroeder (Vol. VI)

- Making Health an Equal Partner to Health Care (2001)

- Adopting the Substance Abuse Goal (1998–1999)

- Program-Related Investments (Vol. V)

- Grantmaking in New Jersey (Vol. V)

- The Foundation's Research Strategies (2000)

- The Foundation's Communications Strategies (2001)

- The Foundation's National Programs (Vol. VIII)

- Responding to Emergencies: 9/11, Bioterrorism, and Natural Disasters (Vol. VII)

- Health, Health Care, and the Robert Wood Johnson Foundation: 1996–2006 (Vol. X)

- Terrance Keenan: An Appreciation (Vol. IX)

Philanthropy

- Public Scrutiny of Foundations and Charities (Vol. IX)

- Partnerships Among Foundations (2001)

- The Local Initiative Funding Partners Program (2000)

Other Topics

- Reflections on the book, *On Doctoring* (Vol. V)

- The National Health and Social Life Survey (1997)

In our introductions to some of the volumes, we have tried to tie the strands together and offer an overview of what the chapters mean for health and health care and/or for philanthropy. We have done this, in particular, in our introductions to the 2001 volume ("Grantmaking Insights from the *Robert Wood Johnson Foundation Anthology*"), *Volume VII* ("Observations on Grantmaking from the *Robert Wood Johnson Foundation Anthology Series*") and Volume IX ("Still Swinging for the Philanthropic Fences?"). Additionally, the *Anthology* series provides a venue for the Foundation's president and CEO to transmit his or her thoughts on substantive matters to a wide audience. Steven Schroeder's foreword to the 1998–1999 volume addressed the core values of the Foundation. Risa Lavizzo-Mourey used the pages of Volume IX to discuss the "five C's" of effective philanthropy and of Volume X to share her ideas on what it takes to make a great foundation.

Taken collectively, the volumes of the *Anthology* present a relatively comprehensive picture of what the Robert Wood Johnson Foundation has done and is doing to improve health and health care. It is important to present this picture, for just as foundations must be financially accountable to the public, so, too, should they be accountable for the programs they fund and activities they carry out. If the *Anthology* serves as a vehicle through which the Foundation is programmatically accountable to the public, then we, as editors, can feel that we have met—in part at least—the challenge that faced us when we talked with Frank Karel in a small Foundation office more than a decade ago.

San Francisco   Stephen L. Isaacs
Princeton, New Jersey   James R. Knickman
May, 2006   Editors

~m~ Acknowledgments

We are grateful to the many people who have made this volume of *The Robert Wood Johnson Foundation Anthology* possible. First and foremost is David Morse, who, in reality, serves as an uncredited third editor. His insights and wisdom improve every chapter. Others at the Foundation also deserve our gratitude: Jessica Morton and Edith Burbank-Schmitt for gathering background materials on the topics covered in this volume; Molly McKaughan for editing all of the chapters; Marian Bass for reviewing drafts of several chapters; Marilyn Ernst for handling administrative matters; Carol Owle, Mary Castria, Carolyn Scholer, and Ellen Coyote for taking care of financial matters; Hope Woodhead and Barbara Sherwood for overseeing the book's distribution; Deborah Malloy and Sherry DeMarchi for serving as liaison between the co-editors; Richard Toth, Lydia Ryba, and Kathleen McGeady for making sure that all references to the Foundation's grants are accurate; Hinda Feige Greenberg, Katherine Flatley, Mary Beth Kren, and Barbara Sergeant for finding reference materials; Anne Weiss, Robert Hughes, and Nancy Barrand for commenting on drafts of individual chapters; and Risa Lavizzo-Mourey for reviewing drafts of all of the volume's chapters.

We also express our appreciation to C. P. Crow for his exceptional editing; Carolyn Shea for her thorough fact checking; and Lauren McIntyre for entering the edits of the manuscript. Debbie Dunn Solomon, Pauline Seitz, and Steven Schroeder reviewed individual chapters, for which we are grateful. We are thankful to the members of the outside review committee—Susan Dentzer, William Morrill, Patricia Patrizi, and Jonathan Showstack—for their usual care in scrutinizing drafts of the chapters and their thoughtful suggestions for improving them. The team at Jossey-Bass—Andy Pasternack, Seth Schwartz, and Kelsey McGee—and Jon Peck of Dovetail Publishing have been key to the publication of the *Anthology,* and their efforts are much appreciated. Finally, we acknowledge the fine work of Elizabeth Dawson who has been an active participant in all stages of the book's preparation and production.

S.L.I. and J.R.K.

To Improve Health and Health Care

Volume X

A Ten-Year Retrospective

1

Health, Health Care, and the Robert Wood Johnson Foundation: A Ten-Year Retrospective, 1996–2006

*Stephen L. Isaacs, James R. Knickman, David J. Morse**

Editors' Introduction

To mark the tenth anniversary issue of *The Robert Wood Johnson Foundation Anthology* series, the editors wanted to take a retrospective look at how health and health care have changed in the decade between 1996 and 2006 and how the Robert Wood Johnson Foundation's approach to the issues has evolved during the same time period. We decided to undertake the task ourselves, in collaboration with David Morse, the Foundation's vice president for communications. Morse has been an active participant in the development, editing, production, and distribution of the *Anthology* series. In addition to investigating how health, health care, and the nation's fourth largest foundation have changed during the decade, we were also curious to find out whether external events had influenced the Foundation's policy agenda, and if so, how.

---

*The authors express their appreciation to Edith Burbank-Schmitt for her research assistance.

Taking 1996 and 2006 as fixed comparison points is somewhat arbitrary. What happened in those years cannot be wholly separated from events that occurred in the preceding years—or, for that matter, the following years. Health care in 1996, for example, cannot be divorced from the attempts at reform that ended a few years earlier. Similarly, the Robert Wood Johnson Foundation's strategies in 2006 reflect decisions made in 2003 when the Foundation adopted an "impact framework" to guide its grantmaking. As we have learned, the Foundation's grantmaking strategies depend to a great extent on the perspectives of the Foundation's president, but they are formulated within the framework developed over many years by the Foundation's staff and trustees.

In a sense, in this chapter we try to answer the question, "How did the nation's largest health foundation approach its mission—to improve the health and health care of all Americans—at two different times set a decade apart?" To find the answers, we first look at how the public and health policy experts saw health and health care issues in 1996, and then again in 2006. We then explore the Foundation's strategic priorities in 1996 and 2006, how they evolved, and why. We then look at the interrelationship between societal concerns and the Foundation's programming to determine, as best we can, if and how the two intersect and what are the implications for health philanthropy.

—ɯ— **1996.** The year that the New York Yankees, show-ing little respect for the hosts of the Centennial Olympics, bested the Atlanta Braves four games to two to win the World Series. The year that *The English Patient* won nine Academy Awards, including best picture. The year that the play *Rent* won the Pulitzer Prize for drama, the rapper Tupac Shakur was gunned down, and Frank McCourt's *Angela's Ashes* was a runaway best-seller. In 1996, Russia and Chechnya signed a cease-fire agreement, a furor over "mad cow disease" broke out in England, and Israel elected Benjamin Netanyahu as its prime minister. That year, Americans lived through a four-month budget crisis that all but para-lyzed the federal government. Later, Congress passed two major pieces of social legislation: Welfare Reform and the Health Insurance Portability and Accountability Act. The economy was strong and was showing the stirrings of the high-tech rally that led some analysts to predict that the Dow Jones average would reach 30,000. In November, America's voters elected Bill Clinton to a second term as president.

That year, both the public and health care professionals focused their attention primarily on managed care, AIDS, and tobacco. Ten years later, the major health issues had changed dramatically, bearing little resem-blance to the issues that had captivated the nation only a decade earlier.

—ɯ— The Shift in Health and Health Care Priorities: 1996–2006

Perhaps the signal health care event of the 1990s was President Clinton's health reform plan and its demise in 1994. The plan's failure unleashed an explosion of managed care plans. In 1996, 73 percent of the insured popu-lation was enrolled in a health maintenance organization or other form of managed care plan, up from 54 percent in 1993.[1] Much of the growth in managed care was in the for-profit sector. Health plans and hospitals vied to shed their nonprofit status and compete as money-making organiza-tions. In the 1990s, for example, the Hospital Corporation of America, a for-profit corporation, became the nation's leading hospital chain by buying nonprofit hospitals throughout the nation. Many formerly non-profit Blue Cross Blue Shield plans joined the stampede to become for-profits.

Two factors drove the rapid growth of managed care. The first was the need to cut the cost of medical services. The second was the desire for better coordination and monitoring of patient care. By integrating delivery systems and paying physicians on a per-patient (rather than a per-procedure) basis, managed care was supposed to offer an incentive to provide appropriate rather than excessive care and therefore save money. Calvin Bland, who in 1996 was the president and chief executive officer of St. Christopher's Hospital for Children in Philadelphia and is currently the chief of staff of the Robert Wood Johnson Foundation, recalls, "The whole focus was on hospital growth through mergers and acquisitions, enrolling people in HMOs, re-engineering hospital services, and cutting costs. It was a time of mergers and megamergers."

By 1996, managed care had succeeded in driving down costs somewhat. But to many, the price of cost-cutting was too high. Members of HMOs found that they could not get referred to specialists easily. They hesitated to visit emergency rooms for fear that their plan would not deem the visit a true emergency and wouldn't cover it. And they were released from hospitals after only a brief stay—in the popular phrase of the day, patients were discharged "quicker and sicker."

While 1996 might have been the high water mark of managed care, it also marked the point where the tide against it picked up force. Congress passed legislation prohibiting "drive-through deliveries," where women who had given birth in a hospital were sent home the next day. Later in the year, Congress passed the Kennedy-Kassebaum bill—or, more formally, the Health Insurance Portability and Accountability Act—which prohibited managed care plans and insurance companies from denying coverage to people with a pre-existing medical condition who changed jobs.

By 1996, AIDS had become an American epidemic and an international calamity, attracting media headlines and drawing the attention of the health community. Between 1981, when the first case was reported, and 1996, more than half a million people over the age of thirteen in the United States had contracted AIDS.[2] The number of new cases reported in 1996—68,000—was nearly double the number reported in 1992.[3] Yet there were signs of hope: many people at risk of contracting HIV were adopting safe sex practices, such as using condoms, and cocktails of antiretroviral drugs offered the prospect of converting AIDS from a death sentence to a chronic condition.

Smoking, too, was on the public's and the health community's mind. Well before 1996, Congress had required warning labels on cigarette packs, prohibited smoking on planes, and banned tobacco commercials on radio and television. By 1996, nearly 1,500 municipalities had enacted clean indoor air restrictions; attorneys general of forty-five states had filed or were preparing to file lawsuits against the tobacco companies; and it looked as if a master settlement agreement between the states and the tobacco companies (which would have settled the suits and committed the tobacco industry to pay significant amounts of money to the states and curtail its cigarette advertising) was within reach.

Although managed care, AIDS, and tobacco dominated the health news and the health policy journals in 1996, other health issues drew attention as well.

- Health insurance. Despite a booming economy and a tight labor market—conditions that one might suppose would have led to increased health insurance coverage—by 1996, the number of uninsured had reached 42 million, a matter of some, but not major, concern in Washington. The next year, Congress passed the State Children's Health Insurance Program, or SCHIP, which offered insurance coverage to poor children throughout the nation.

- Abortion and teenage pregnancy. Both of these reproductive health issues remained highly controversial and newsworthy.

- Drug abuse. Although substance abuse appeared to be less of a crisis than it had in the 1980s, the availability and use of illegal drugs remained a concern.

- End-of-life care. Sparked in part by a Robert Wood Johnson Foundation-funded study that found that physicians

routinely ignored the wishes of dying patients, the care
of patients toward the end of their lives was becoming an
important health issue.[4]

Fast forward to 2006. Managed care has been largely transformed
from a tiger to a pussycat. The restrictive systems that could, in theory,
better manage patients' care and hold down costs were replaced by more
open systems where cost saving was not the dominant feature.

Perhaps as a result of the changes in managed care, health care costs
have gone through the roof. Premiums have risen by around 10 percent
a year between 2000 and 2005, and fewer businesses—especially small
ones—provide health insurance for their employees.[5] Sixty percent of
firms offered their employees coverage in 2005, down from 69 percent
in 2000.[6] When employers do provide health insurance coverage, premiums are increasingly borne by employees (in 2005, employees paid
nearly $1,100 more a year for family coverage, on average, than they
did in 1996).[7] "The affordability of health insurance is a cyclical issue,"
said Paul Ginsburg, president of the Center for Studying Health System
Change. "In 1996, managed care had slowed the rise in health insurance
premiums, and premiums had actually flattened out. By 2006, costs had
risen again, and a lot of people were afraid they wouldn't be able to
afford health insurance premiums."

At the same time, the number of uninsured has spiraled steadily
upward, reaching nearly 46 million in 2005.[8] This upward spiral strains
safety net providers such as public hospitals, free clinics, and community
health centers, and it has serious health consequences as sick people delay
seeking medical care until their illnesses become too serious to ignore and
they then go to hospital emergency rooms for treatment. Health insurance
coverage has emerged as the number one issue in labor contract negotiations. Medicaid, the backbone of insurance coverage for poor people, is in
serious trouble as both federal and state governments seek to cut back their
Medicaid budgets, which in many states have become unsustainable.

Even as the cost of medical care and the number of uninsured have
risen to previously unthinkable levels, and underserved people living in
inner cities and rural areas *still* have trouble finding a doctor, few in the

federal government seem willing to address the issue of coverage. The only major change has been the addition of a prescription drug benefit to Medicare, which took effect on January 1, 2006, to the confusion of seniors baffled by a bewildering array of choices. Beyond Washington, some states, most recently Massachusetts, and cities have passed or are considering legislation to insure all their residents, but whether these programs are affordable remains a question.

Health care coverage now is a bitterly contested, often partisan issue in Washington. Some analysts and politicians, contending that health insurance should be a private sector responsibility, back "consumer-driven health plans" managed by insurance companies. Others argue that it is government's responsibility to assure that all members of society have health insurance—that it is costly and inefficient to leave something as important as the nation's health to market forces. The issue has become so highly politicized that few, if any, analysts see major change coming in the near future. "At least the system hasn't fallen apart," said John Lumpkin, former director of the Illinois Department of Public Health and currently a senior vice president at the Robert Wood Johnson Foundation. "Without a major transforming event, however, little is likely to happen at the federal level. At most, the system will undergo small evolutionary changes."

Not only is access to health insurance precarious, but the public feels more vulnerable, its insecurity having been fed by September 11th, the anthrax attacks that followed the next month, and the threat of a bird flu pandemic. After September 11th, and the anthrax attacks, Congress appropriated funds to enable the governmental public health system to better prepare for a bioterror attack and, in 2006, to strengthen the public health system's capacity to cope with an avian flu epidemic. But whether the nation's public health system—which the Institute of Medicine characterized as being "in disarray" in 1988 and again in 2002—is up to the challenge posed by the new threats is not known.[9]

While tobacco remains the nation's number one cause of preventable death, obesity may have eclipsed it as a health concern. The percentage of overweight and obese individuals rose from 45 percent in 1990 to 52 percent in 1996 (when the problem was barely discussed) to 66 percent in 2005. Obesity causes heart attacks, strokes, and diabetes, among other illnesses. It is increasingly prevalent in children, who are likely to grow up to be obese adults. "It is clear that childhood obesity is becoming a hot button political issue," said Mark DiCamillo, director of the California-based Field Institute.

Obesity, smoking, unhealthy environments, high stress, and lack of health insurance hit the poor harder than the rich, and blacks and Hispanics harder than whites. Racial and ethnic minorities and people of lower socioeconomic class have far higher rates of heart attacks, strokes, some cancers, cavities, hypertension, and diabetes than do the white majority. While the nation was certainly aware of racial, ethnic, and class differences in health status in 1996, these were not a dominant issue. After Hurricane Katrina graphically exposed an American society of haves and have-nots, reducing racial and ethnic disparities in health moved somewhat higher on—though nowhere near the top of—the nation's policy agenda.

Ever since the Institute of Medicine's 1999 report *To Err is Human* estimated that as many as 98,000 people die annually from illnesses contracted in the hospital, improving the quality of medical care has attracted more attention in the health policy community. The National Committee for Quality Assurance's work to develop quality standards for managed care organizations in the 1990s has expanded into wide-ranging efforts to measure quality and to hold health plans, hospitals, and physicians accountable for the quality of their services. The Center for Studying Health System Change's Paul Ginsburg said that the focus on quality is far different in 2006 from the focus of 1996: "In 1996, it was organizations like the American Medical Association arguing that restrictions on care would harm quality. Now there is a different perspective: quality refers to real failings in the way health care is delivered." He added, however, "Quality is of concern to policy makers, but it hasn't crossed into the public's consciousness yet."

The most significant changes in health and health care between 1996 and 2006 can be briefly summarized:

- In 1996, the changing health care system—restrictive managed care plans, for-profit health plans and hospitals, takeovers of local hospitals by big national chains, mergers of big health care systems—worried the public and policy makers. By 2006, the changes had run their course; employees tended to enroll in less restrictive managed care plans; and the concerns about managed care had largely faded.

- In 1996, costs appeared to be coming under control, mainly because managed care had clamped a lid on them. By 2006, they were out of control again, increasing at a steady 10 percent a year.

- In 1996, the number of uninsured Americans stood at 42 million, but lack of health insurance coverage was not attracting much attention. As a result of high premiums, in the 2000s, businesses cut back on buying health insurance for their employees. By 2006, the number of uninsured was rising at one million people a year, the number of uninsured individuals reached 46 million, and health insurance coverage was again back on the national political agenda.

- In 1996, Medicaid and Medicare hardly made the news. By 2006, both federal and state governments were looking for ways to cut back their Medicaid expenditures, which in some states had surpassed 30 percent of the annual budget. The enrollment problems with the Medicare prescription drug plan made the nightly news with fair regularity.

- In 1996, the governmental public health system was weak and ineffective, but hardly anybody noticed. By 2006, September 11th, the anthrax attacks, and the potential for a bird flu pandemic had raised awareness of the need for a stronger governmental public health system as a first line of defense against bioterrorism and the spread of infectious diseases.

- In 1996, AIDS was a national tragedy, very much on the public's mind. By 2006, though it had reached epidemic proportions internationally, changing sexual practices had

reduced the incidence of AIDS in the United States, and
pharmacological advances made it possible for HIV-positive
Americans to live for many years.

■ In 1996, almost nobody was talking about obesity as a
national health problem. In 2006, newspapers, radio, and
television bombarded the public, and awareness of obesity
as a problem was high. At the same time, tobacco, a major
issue in 1996, receded somewhat. (Even though tobacco
remained the nation's number one killer in 2006, prevalence
of smoking was at an all time low and youth smoking was the
lowest in nearly three decades.)

—ɷ— The Robert Wood Johnson Foundation: 1996–2006

Foundations do not make a fresh start every year, every decade, or with
every change of leadership. They are guided and bounded by their mission, their history, and their past grant-making patterns. In both 1996 and
2006, the Foundation was well along on a course that had been set initially
by its first board of trustees in 1972 and was guided by priorities that had
been developing for decades. Working within those limitations, and cog-
nizant of the social, economic, and political circumstances that affected the
nation's health, the Foundation made two critical strategic shifts.

The first shift, made gradually in the early and mid-1990s under the
leadership of the Foundation's president, Steven Schroeder, was expanding the Foundation's scope of activities to include not just *health care*
but *health* as well. Influenced by a powerful literature demonstrating the
social, economic, and behavioral determinants of health status and the
experience of five years of tobacco-control and other substance-control
programs, the Foundation in 1996 was poised to recognize publicly that
addressing the root causes of poor health was as important as addressing
the lack of access to medical care. The president's message to the board
in January, 1997, urged it to give *health* a priority equal to that of *health
care*. By 1999, the Foundation had reorganized into two divisions, one

devoted to improving health care and the other to improving health. The latter built on and provided a conceptual underpinning for the Foundation's grant making in areas such as addiction prevention and treatment, childhood obesity, and supportive housing for homeless people.

The Foundation's approach focused on several big ideas—access to care, chronic illness, substance abuse—and concentrated resources where they might be needed, even on short notice.

In contrast, the second strategic shift, which began shortly after Risa Lavizzo-Mourey assumed the Foundation's presidency in 2003, took a more targeted approach, honing in on a limited number of objectives whose impact could be measured quantitatively. With the adoption of an "impact framework," the Foundation established a "portfolio" of grants targeting ten priority areas (later reduced to eight)—some of which sought to improve the behaviors, lifestyles, and conditions that lead to better health and others of which aimed at expanding access to, and improving the quality of, health care—and set specific, measurable strategic objectives for each of them. It also established three other portfolios: one that addressed issues affecting vulnerable populations, a second that focused on building human capital, and a third that sought to nurture new and promising ideas.

The change in the Foundation's thinking between 1996 and 2006 can be illustrated by examining three critical areas: encouraging healthy behaviors and lifestyles; expanding access to medical care; and improving the quality of care.

Encouraging Healthy Behaviors and Lifestyles: From Tobacco to Obesity

In 1991, it was hardly a secret that smoking caused cancer, heart disease, and stroke, among other fatal illnesses. When the Foundation took the step of making tobacco control a priority that year, it was able to do what it had done well in the past: help shape an emerging field.[10] Its grant making began somewhat timidly, with a relatively small grant to look at ways to reduce teenage smoking in four communities. Gradually, the Foundation became emboldened, and by 1996 it was in the process of developing a multi-pronged strategy to reduce smoking whose components were: (1) tobacco-policy research; (2) advocacy aimed at counteracting the tobacco industry's influence and informing policy change; (3) demonstration programs that put research into practice; (4) dissemination of tobacco-cessation standards; and (5) communications activities. In addition, the Foundation's president used the prestige of his office to keep the issue high on the nation's health agenda. Michael Pertschuk, co-founder of the Advocacy Institute and former chairman of the Federal Trade Commission, noted that the Foundation had taken on "the fundamental political dimension of the problem. It was a unique strategic intervention in the public health field that will serve as a model for years to come."[11]

From its experience in tobacco-control programs of the 1990s, the Foundation gained knowledge that it is applying to other areas. One lesson is the value of bringing to bear a broad range of approaches—what the health policy writer James Bornemeier called "a sustained flow of financial resources to all corners of the field."[12] Another is the importance of policy change. "The Foundation found a niche that government agencies could not fill, especially policy research and demonstration programs," said James Marks, senior vice president of the Robert Wood Johnson Foundation. "We learned that when a grant for services ends, the program often ends, but policy change persists." A third lesson is that a foundation can play a role beyond simply making grants. "Our prominence in the field meant that we were often a convener—a switchboard, as it were," Marks continued.

Recognizing the sustained drop in smoking rates and the need to address other threats to the nation's health, in 2003 the Foundation decided to gradually phase out its funding of tobacco-control initiatives while working with its grantees to maintain the gains that they had made. By 2006, the foundation's tobacco-control activities had moved principally to supporting efforts to reduce smoking in public places and to decreasing the demand for tobacco.

Barely on the radar screen in 1996, obesity is, in 2006, a public health threat that has captured the public's attention. The Foundation came to embrace reducing obesity as a priority somewhat circuitously. In 2001, it made healthy communities and healthy lifestyles a priority area. Focusing first on encouraging physical activity, the Foundation awarded grants that helped communities become friendlier to walking, biking, and other forms of exercise.[13] By 2003, however, as obesity became a major public health issue, the Foundation made halting the upward trend in childhood obesity one of its strategic objectives, and added nutrition to the work it had been doing to promote physical activity.

Like tobacco in the early and mid-1990s, obesity is an emerging field whose direction the Foundation may help shape. The similarities between tobacco and obesity are unmistakable: both involve harmful personal behaviors and both fall hardest upon people of limited means. There are also differences: nicotine is an addictive substance, while foods have not been shown to be physiologically addictive; tobacco had a villain, while no such obvious heavy has appeared in the nutrition or physical activity areas; and while second-hand smoke aroused people whose health was affected by the smoking of others, there is no similar rallying point around obesity.

Building on the similarities and adapting the approach it employed in its tobacco-control initiatives, the Foundation is planning to use a broad range of approaches to reach the goal of halting the increase in childhood obesity by 2015. These include building the science base, funding pilot programs in schools and communities, producing information for the media and the public, convening activists, and providing information for policy makers. The specific directions of the Foundation's approach toward childhood obesity are still emerging, and tangible national indicators of success or failure will probably not emerge for years.

Expanding Health Insurance Coverage: From State and Local to National Approaches

Over the years, the Foundation has oscillated between two different approaches to expanding coverage for the uninsured.[14]

The first approach, an incremental one that tries to bring about change at the state and local levels, was dominant in 1996. In part, this resulted from the Foundation's role in health reform. In 1992 and 1993, as President Bill Clinton's plan to reform health insurance was being developed and debated, the Foundation and its grantees were a source of information on health policy. Foundation staff members helped organize a series of meetings with Hillary Clinton to help explain the proposals for national reform. Some people were critical of the Foundation for playing what they viewed as a partisan role. Stung by criticism that it had taken sides in the debate, the Foundation pulled back.

Instead of promoting national health care reform, it adopted instead a posture of encouraging incremental change at the state and community levels while also showing a willingness to support existing federal programs. Commenting on the Foundation's move from the front lines of the political debate, the Foundation's president, Risa Lavizzo-Mourey, said, "Up to the early 1990s, the Foundation had never been in the crosshairs of a political debate, even with its work in AIDS in the 1980s. We learned how politicized the issue of coverage had become and, for us, the importance of being nonpartisan. We also learned that we can be most effective if we are neutral conveners."

In 1996, the Foundation's efforts to help states and localities expand health insurance was characterized by a program called Communities In Charge. Looking to emulate an apparently successful program in the Tampa Bay area of Florida that raised the local sales tax in order to finance a managed-care plan for uninsured people, the Foundation was planning a program that would support fourteen communities' plans to provide insurance coverage to their uninsured.[15]

The Foundation was also able to support the federal government through a program called Covering Kids, which let parents of poor children in fifteen states know that their kids might be eligible for Medicaid and attempted to simplify the application and approval process. Shortly after the Foundation authorized funds for Covering Kids, Congress passed the State Children's Health Insurance Program, or SCHIP, that made health insurance available for poor children. Taking advantage of the new federal legislation, the Foundation dramatically increased its support of Covering Kids, expanded the program to all fifty states, and developed a major media campaign to accompany it.

The second approach was to promote action to expand health insurance coverage at the national level. By 2006, the pendulum had largely swung back as the Foundation recognized that major change, if it happens at all, is likely to come from Washington. "Incrementalism is the second best solution," said the Foundation senior program officer Nancy Barrand. "How can we settle for second best?"

The return of the pendulum began in 1999 when the Foundation convened a meeting of a group of Washington-based policy experts and activists from all over the political spectrum concerned with the problem of the uninsured. Called "the strange bedfellows," the group agreed on the need to cover the uninsured; it continues to meet and look for ways to do it. By 2003, the strange bedfellows meetings had led the Foundation to organize the first Cover the Uninsured Week—a large-scale public relations campaign designed to remind the nation that millions of people are uninsured and that the lack of insurance harms their health. Cover the Uninsured Weeks have been an annual event since then.

In 2006, one of the Foundation's strategic objectives is enactment of a national policy ensuring stable and affordable coverage for all by the year 2010. It does not endorse any single path toward reaching that goal, however. "While we know where we want to go—stable and affordable coverage for all—we don't take a position on how to get there," Lavizzo-Mourey said. "The issue is highly politicized, and there is no consensus on a solution. I doubt that there is even a consensus among our staff and board."

While many people give the Foundation credit for sticking with the issue, twenty years of Foundation attention to it appears to have yielded little tangible success. If the Foundation's work to expand health insurance coverage taught it to temper its expectations, its experience in a related area—cost containment—was positively humbling. In 1996, the Foundation was trying to reduce the cost of health care, but it found that in a trillion dollar-plus health economy, it had little leverage. "One of the lessons we internalized from the 1990s has to do with health care costs," Risa Lavizzo-Mourey said. "We've come to understand what we can and cannot do. Here, the system is dependent on reimbursement. We've learned to avoid areas where we have few effective levers."

Improving the Quality of Care:
From Scattered Programs to Systemic Change

Without using the word "quality" as an objective, the Robert Wood Johnson Foundation was doing a great deal to improve the quality of care of people in 1996, especially the care provided to people with chronic illnesses. For example, it supported the National Committee for Quality Assurance, the National Quality Forum, the Institute for Healthcare Improvement, and *The Dartmouth Atlas of Health Care*.[16] And it developed programs to give chronically ill people the option of paying friends and relatives, rather than agencies, to take care of them;[17] to connect nursing schools and nursing homes in order to improve the quality of care provided in nursing homes;[18] and, most prominently, to improve the care given to dying people.[19]

In 1995, amid great fanfare, the Foundation released the disappointing results of a study it had funded called SUPPORT (the Study to Understand Prognoses and Preferences for Outcomes and Risks of Treatment).[20] The findings from SUPPORT revealed that physicians and hospitals routinely ignored the wishes of dying patients and their families. In light of these discouraging findings, the Foundation decided to mount a campaign directed at improving the care that people receive toward the end of their lives. In 1996, staff members at the Foundation were preparing the campaign, which got under way the next year.

As in the case of tobacco control, the Foundation entered a field in which there was already a lot of interest and took a multipronged approach to shaping it—funding palliative care programs at major medical centers, medical and nursing curricula improvement, coalitions of advocates, articles in leading medical and nursing journals, and a Bill Moyers PBS series on end-of-life care called *On Our Own Terms,* which was seen by an estimated nineteen million viewers. In 2003, as it was reconsidering its priorities, the Foundation concluded that, like its tobacco programs, its end-of-life programs had largely achieved what they had set out to do, and decided to phase out its support. As of 2006, the Foundation had ended most of its end-of-life grant making, with the exception of the Center to Advance Palliative Care, which it continues to support in concert with other major funders.

By 2006, building on its work over the past decade, the Foundation had made improving the quality of care for people with chronic illness one of its strategic priorities. As one example, in 1996, the Foundation was supporting the Group Health Cooperative of Puget Sound, a Seattle-based health maintenance organization, in its development of a new model of providing high-quality care to people with chronic illnesses. This led to the Foundation's funding, in 1998, the Improving Chronic Illness Care program that tested the chronic care model in a number of different locations.[21] Though the chronic care model requires a rethinking of the way in which medical care is organized, by 2006, it was gaining increasing recognition as an effective way of treating people with a wide variety of chronic illnesses.

The Foundation has gone well beyond its stated goal of trying to improve quality of care only for chronically ill people, and, in practice, is trying to improve the quality of care of patients generally, whatever their medical condition. Between 2001 and 2006, it authorized at least seven major programs focused directly on quality improvement; commissioned Institute of Medicine reports on the topic; and created an eponymous team to oversee its quality improvement efforts. It has funded the work of the Institute for Healthcare Improvement, for example, to reduce medical errors. Moreover, the concern about quality infuses many of the Foundation's programs, such as its nursing and addiction prevention and treatment programs.

—w— Conclusion

The Robert Wood Johnson Foundation's board and staff continually grapple with the question of how the organization can best fulfill its mission of improving the health and health care of all Americans—a question whose answer is complicated by the recognition that while the Foundation is a major force in health philanthropy, it is only a tiny player in a trillion dollar-plus health economy.

In 1996, the Foundation's approach was articulated by three broadly ambitious goals—increasing access to care, improving the care of people with chronic illness, and reducing the harm caused by substance abuse. To achieve them, it gave the health side of its mission as much importance as the health care side and devoted substantial resources to comprehensive approaches to addressing a few critical health issues such as smoking and end-of-life care.

In 2003, the Foundation developed an impact framework, which continues to guide its programming in 2006. The impact framework takes a more targeted approach—establishing measurable short-term, medium-term, and long-term targets for eight priority areas and allocating funds in an equitable manner among them. At the same time, the Foundation continues to give high priority to improving the health care workforce, finding better ways to provide care to the underserved, and seeking innovative new ideas.

Risa Lavizzo-Mourey has observed, "As a result of the changes that began in the mid-1990s, we were forced to question our approaches to social change." The impact framework articulates the Robert Wood Johnson Foundation's approach to social change in the health and health care fields in 2006, just as the three goals did in 1996. Neither approach is better or worse, right or wrong. They are, however, different, and represent the ways that the Foundation's leadership, working within the framework of the institution's history and past priorities, seeks to achieve its mission.

The Foundation's approach to social change is based in part—and only in part—on its attempt to be responsive to the external environment. A foundation that is overresponsive to changing public opinion risks becoming faddish, yet one that ignores the concerns of the public and policy makers risks being out of touch. Striking a balance requires a deft touch.

Over the years, staff members and trustees have learned that some of the Foundation's most effective programs have been those in which the Foundation has entered fields as they were emerging and then shaped the direction they took. The most obvious examples are tobacco control and end-of-life care in the 1990s, but earlier programs—nurse practitioners and emergency medical services, for example—buttress the point. Some of the Foundation's current programming—for example, strengthening the public health system and reducing childhood obesity—builds on issues that are now viewed as critical to the nation's health and well-being. These are issues that emerged between 1996 and 2006 that concern the public and have captured its attention and whose direction the Foundation may be able to affect.

However, entering emerging fields and working to shape them explains only part of the Foundation's strategies. While the Foundation has learned that it needs to be responsive to the external environment, it has also learned that it must remain true to its principles, even when they may not be in sync with prevailing wisdom. Some of its current objectives, therefore, represent areas that are not high on the public agenda. Improving the quality of care and reducing disparities did not resonate loudly with the public in 1996 and still do not. But they are important to the Robert Wood Johnson Foundation. Making issues such as these a priority gives the Foundation an opportunity to play a leadership role and to help make them more prominent. Or, simply, to promote values it believes are important for the nation's health.

Notes

1. Kaiser Commission on Medicaid and the Uninsured. *Trends and Indicators in the Changing Health Care Marketplace,* Exhibit 3.5. Menlo Park, Calif.: Kaiser Family Foundation, 2005. (www.kkf.org/insurance/7031/ti2004-2-3.cfm)
2. CDC. "HIV and AIDS Cases Reported Through December 1996." *HIV/AIDS Surveillance Report,* 1997, 8(2).
3. CDC. "HIV and AIDS—United States, 1981–2000." *Morbidity and Mortality Weekly Report,* June 1, 2001.
4. Lynn, J. "Unexpected Returns: Insights from SUPPORT." *To Improve Health and Health Care 2001: The Robert Wood Johnson Foundation Anthology.* San Francisco: Jossey-Bass, 2001.
5. Kaiser Family Foundation and Health Research and Educational Trust. *Employer Health Benefits: 2005. Summary of Findings.* Menlo Park, Calif.: Kaiser Family Foundation, 2006.
6. Ibid.
7. Kaiser Commission on Medicaid and the Uninsured. *Trends and Indicators in the Changing Health Care Marketplace,* Exhibit 3.5. Menlo Park, Calif.: Kaiser Family Foundation, 2005. (www.kkf.org/insurance/7031/print-sec3.cfm)

8. U.S. Census Bureau. *Income Stable, Poverty Increases, Percentage of Americans without Health Care Unchanged.* August 30, 2005. (www. census.gov/press-release/www/releases/archives/income_wealth/005647. html)

9. Institute of Medicine. *The Future of the Public's Health in the 21st Century.* Washington, D.C.: National Academies Press, 2002.

10. Isaacs, S. L., and Knickman, J. R. "Field Building: Lessons from the Robert Wood Johnson Foundation's Anthology Series." *Health Affairs,* 2005, *24*(4), 1161–1165.

11. Bornemeier, J. "Taking on Tobacco: The Robert Wood Johnson Foundation's Assault on Smoking." *To Improve Health and Health Care, Vol. VIII: The Robert Wood Johnson Foundation Anthology.* San Francisco: Jossey-Bass, 2005, p. 21.

12. Ibid.

13. Robert Wood Johnson Foundation. *Lessons Learned: Promoting Physical Activity at the Community Level.* Grant Results Special Report, September 2005. (http://www.rwjf.org/files/publications/ LessonsLearned_PhysicalActivity_GRR.pdf)

14. Rosenblatt, R. "The Robert Wood Johnson Foundation's Efforts to Cover the Uninsured." *To Improve Health and Health Care, Vol. IX: The Robert Wood Johnson Foundation Anthology.* San Francisco: Jossey-Bass, 2006.

15. See Chapter Four in this volume.

16. See Chapter Two in this volume.

17. Benjamin, A. E., and Snyder, R. E. "Consumer Choice in Long-Term Care." *To Improve Health and Health Care, Vol. V: The Robert Wood Johnson Foundation Anthology.* San Francisco: Jossey-Bass, 2002.

18. Bronner, E. "The Teaching Nursing Home Program." *To Improve Health and Health Care, Vol. VII: The Robert Wood Johnson Foundation Anthology.* San Francisco: Jossey-Bass, 2004.

19. Bronner, E. "The Foundation's End-of-Life Programs: Changing the American Way of Death." *To Improve Health and Health Care, Vol. VI: The Robert Wood Johnson Foundation Anthology.* San Francisco: Jossey-Bass, 2003.

20. Lynn, J. "Unexpected Returns: Insights from SUPPORT." *To Improve Health and Health Care 1997: The Robert Wood Johnson Foundation Anthology.* San Francisco: Jossey-Bass, 1997.

21. See Chapter Three in this volume.

Quality of Care

2

The Dartmouth Atlas of Health Care

Carolyn Newbergh

Editors' Introduction

This year's volume of the *Anthology* features two chapters that examine the Foundation's efforts to improve the quality of medical care. In the following chapter, Irene Wielawski looks at the chronic care model, a systematic way of treating patients with chronic conditions. In this chapter, Carolyn Newbergh, a freelance writer specializing in health care, discusses *The Dartmouth Atlas of Health Care* and the other work of Dr. Jack Wennberg highlighting the capricious way that patients receive medical care depending on where they live.

Wennberg and his colleagues at the Center for Evaluative Clinical Sciences at Dartmouth Medical School have demonstrated that physicians in many communities are providing too much care that has little, if any, impact on health, and may even be harmful. They make the case that the health care system could save a considerable amount of money without sacrificing quality if excessive and unnecessary care were eliminated. At the same time, they have shown that many physicians do not deliver the kinds of basic care that are known to be beneficial to patients.

While Wennberg's work on variation of health care has been widely recognized by health policy experts, it has had little influence on medical practice. The same is true of the chronic care model discussed in Chapter 3. This lack of acceptance points up the challenge of changing behavior and systems in ways that will provide high-quality care to patients and allocate limited health care resources wisely.

—ɯ—**I**t turns out that in health care, as in real estate, it all boils down to location, location, location. This doesn't mean you have to live near a world-class medical center to have the best shot at surviving a heart attack. What it does mean, surprisingly, is that where you live is an indicator of just how often you will see your doctor or a specialist, how many MRIs and other diagnostic tests you will have, and when your doctor will tell you that you need an operation. That's the conclusion of a New Hampshire physician, epidemiologist, and professor, John "Jack" Wennberg, who has spent more than thirty-three years examining what's going on in exam rooms and at hospital bedsides, building an ever-more sophisticated understanding of just how crucial geography is to the health care we all receive.

Along the way, Wennberg has shot gaping holes into some tenets of conventional medical wisdom. He dismisses the notion that more medical care is better medical care, that more diagnostic testing is in your best interest, and that the doctor almost always knows best. What's really true, he says, is this:

- More health care can actually mean worse health care.
- There is enormous variation in communities throughout the nation in the kind and amount of health care services being given, with people in some areas receiving more than twice as much in terms of office visits, specialist care, testing, and hospitalization as residents of other areas.
- Much of this difference comes about because doctors have their own practice styles.
- The over-supply of hospital beds, specialists, and diagnostic testing facilities creates demand for these services.
- There is great uncertainty about how best to treat many conditions.
- Much of the excess unwarranted care could be reduced if patients were better informed about their treatment choices.

—m— Making the Case for Geography as Destiny

Wennberg's work, much of it supported by the Robert Wood Johnson Foundation, has revealed some stunning facts. Medicare spends 2.5 times as much on its Miami enrollees as it does on those in Minneapolis—for no good reason and with apparently worse outcomes. The $50,000 more that Medicare spends on Miamians than it does on patients in Minneapolis is "equivalent to a new Lexus GS 400 with all the trimmings," Wennberg wrote provocatively.[1]

The 73-year-old Wennberg, something of a lone wolf and a maverick all these years, has been on a bit of a crusade since he and his colleague Alan Gittelsohn noticed something peculiar back in the early 1970s: kids in one Vermont town were having their tonsils removed in droves, but next door, where Wennberg lived with his wife and four children, hardly any tonsils were being pulled. (Wennberg's own tonsils were removed twice when he was a child, he revealed with a raised eyebrow, and the reason remains something of a mystery to him.) This kind of marked disparity popped up all over the state, so that if you mapped it, a crazy-quilt pattern emerged with no reason for the differences. This was particularly telling in a small state whose residents at the time were demographically alike. Could the children in one town have more tonsillitis than those in the next town over, year after year? Wennberg and Gittelsohn found that that wasn't so. Could it be that parents in one town preferred having their kids undergo tonsillectomies while parents a town away didn't? Not likely.

In 1973, Wennberg and Gittelsohn told this story in the pages of *Science* when no other peer-reviewed journal would publish it. In their landmark study, they linked patients' zip codes to insurance claims records, dividing Vermont into thirteen service areas, based on where people received hospital care. Then, introducing a method they called "small area analysis," they examined rates of tonsillectomies and eight other operations that were adjusted for differences in age. What they discovered was striking: There was a 66 percent chance that a Vermont child living in the service area with the most tonsillectomies would have the operation by age 20, while the likelihood was just 16 to 22 percent in five nearby towns. Similar variations popped up in the eight other common surgeries studied, such as appendectomy, gall bladder, and prostate surgery—variations that could not be attributed to age or different illness levels.[2]

They went on to find, in other studies, the same kind of geographical patterns for the nine common types of surgeries in Maine and then throughout the New England states.[3] In one Maine city, for instance, they discovered that hysterectomies were so frequent that if they continued at the same pace, "70 percent of the women there will have had the operation by the time they reach the age of 75." The authors observed, "In one city surgeons appear to be enthusiastic about hysterectomy; in the other, they appear to be skeptical of its value."[4] Similarly, some hospital service areas had four times as many prostatectomies as others.

It followed that where more health care was being given, more health care dollars were being spent, both in private insurance and in Medicare. Per-capita spending on hospital care in Boston, for instance, was $324 in 1975 while $225 was spent in Providence, $153 in New Haven, and $120 in Hanover, New Hampshire—all communities where care was delivered in prestigious teaching hospitals that one might presume to be of similar quality. The authors pointed out that although third parties, consumers, and the government contributed the same amount for health coverage in these areas, more money was actually being lavished on patients in the high-use areas. In other words, money was being shifted or transferred in what amounted to a subsidy of high-use areas by the low-use ones.

To top off the string of bad news, Wennberg and Gittelsohn found that there was no apparent health benefit to all this extra care. Those who received more health care services did not seem to be healthier or to live longer. A closer examination of this point would come years later.

Why was this pattern of treatment occurring? From these early studies, some theories emerged. Communities that delivered the most health care service tended to have more hospitals and specialists, leading the authors to conclude that greater supply inclines doctors to fill the beds or the appointment slots—because of pressure, incentives, or purely subliminal reasons. But the authors suggested that the biggest determining factor for the variations was the practice style of the doctors themselves. Where an operation was being performed more frequently, more of the doctors in that area were approaching the condition aggressively instead of taking a wait-and-see or medication approach, producing a "surgical signature."

They also found a surprising amount of uncertainty about what the best course of treatment was in many instances. "It seems that the procedures whose rates vary the most are the ones whose risk and benefits are least well established in the medical profession," they wrote. And they posited that the different physician opinions were often a sign that not all doctors were incorporating "new medical knowledge" into their practices. In too many other instances, medical knowledge was not developed enough and more clinical studies were needed to determine what was the best approach to, say, lower back pain or how extensive breast cancer surgery should be. "For many common illnesses, well-designed studies to test alternative forms of therapy have not been done," they wrote. "Many diagnostic and therapeutic techniques are adopted or discarded on the basis of fashion or a physician's personal experience rather than on more reliable grounds." They called for the government to promote outcomes research to clear up the many uncertainties.

These controversial studies bucked the tide of mainstream medical practice and were a lot for the medical world to swallow. It didn't react well. After all, the message was that doctors, who pride themselves on practicing a profession rooted in science, weren't basing most of their decisions on science or clinical trials that had proved particular treatments to be highly effective. Rather, the authors were saying, doctors were more inclined to recommend an operation because of the number of hospital beds that were available or because they worked in a medical group that was aggressive about certain procedures. The many critics said that the studies' findings of extreme variations in care must be wrong, that the differences probably weren't so pronounced, and that there were likely obvious but overlooked explanations for the disparities.

"It used to be you couldn't go to a medical meeting without being heckled, or maybe I should say without encountering people who were really pissed off," says Wennberg, interviewed in his Hanover, New Hampshire, office on the Dartmouth College campus where he is a professor of medicine.

But Wennberg believed that he was on to something and persevered. In other research, he showed that Boston had 60 percent more hospital beds and hospitalized far more patients per capita than New Haven did—a striking illustration of the impact of supply on utilization, given that the two communities boast similar well-regarded medical systems. Although mortality rates were about the same for New Haven and Boston, the costs for hospitalization in Boston were almost double what they were in New Haven.[5]

With the nation's health care costs spiraling ever higher, Wennberg insisted that instead of more and more health care, what we really needed to focus on was the quality of the health care, or value. Then, if the care that was of no value could be reduced or eliminated, a huge cost savings would result. Wennberg's team of researchers estimated in 2003 that by lowering the spending level in high-use regions to that of the low-use regions, Medicare could save about 29 percent a year—which translates to approximately $59 billion—and thus freeing up money for prescription drug benefits for Medicare recipients, strengthening the Medicare system itself, delivering health care to the uninsured, or even meeting other social needs such as improving education.[6]

It would be a long, tough, single-minded fight, but the Robert Wood Johnson Foundation believed, too, that Wennberg was on to something that could make a difference. The Foundation lent crucial financial support to what may be his most ambitious endeavor, *The Dartmouth Atlas of Health Care.* A series of reports and maps that depict variations in health care nationwide over time, the *Atlas* extended Wennberg's early findings from small area analysis in New England to the whole nation, breaking down how Medicare was functioning and finding similar patterns in the private health care market. The Foundation's nearly $10 million in grants over thirteen years also supported further analysis of what was beneath the variations and helped get the word out that something was very wrong.

—w— The Robert Wood Johnson Foundation and the Dartmouth Atlas

It may have seemed as if the whole world was aligned against Wennberg and trying to resist his messages during the 1970s and 1980s, but there were many in the health care trenches treating patients who thought that he was hitting the nail squarely on the head. One of them was Steven Schroeder, a young doctor at George Washington University, who would be a champion of Wennberg's work at the Robert Wood Johnson Foundation when he became its president in 1990. By then, Schroeder had been tracking Wennberg's work for about fifteen years and noting the high caliber of researchers he gathered around him.

"I felt the same way he did," Schroeder said in an interview. "I had done similar work on a smaller scale at George Washington before I knew about Jack's work. My research showed a 17-fold difference in use and costs of lab tests by internists at our medical clinic. I found there was a huge spectrum between people who ordered lots of expensive tests and procedures and those who didn't. I noticed this in my clinical rotation, too. People had very, very different practice styles and the expense of the style didn't correlate into better outcomes."

Wennberg approached the Foundation in the early 1990s to ask for funding to support his efforts to help with the possible implementation of the Clinton health care reform plan. As envisioned at the time, regional insurance purchasing cooperatives might be asked to manage health care resources. Wennberg proposed to show state governments or the cooperatives how to use small area data in managing health care reform. He also had a sketchy idea of producing a series of reports in an "atlas format" that would describe oversupply in the system and the demographics of health before reform as well as track change as it occurred.

The request fell on receptive ears. Wennberg, whose earlier work had been supported largely by the federal government, the John A. Hartford Foundation, and the Commonwealth Fund, received a three-year $2.3 million grant from the Robert Wood Johnson Foundation in 1994. It covered the cost of acquiring and analyzing data as well as preparing policy-relevant reports. Former Foundation executive vice president Lewis

Sandy, now an executive vice president with United HealthCare, recalls that this first grant was "less specifically started as furthering a Foundation objective and more as a project that really was betting on a strong horse and the track record of Jack Wennberg and his team."

When President Clinton's efforts to pass a health plan collapsed, the project was reconfigured to extend the small area analysis Wennberg and his associates had done for New England to the 306 hospital-referral regions and 3,436 "geographically distinct hospital service areas" his team had identified nationwide. The project would analyze how health care resources were distributed and used in each area, all based on Medicare claims data for hospital and outpatient care as well as some private insurance sources. A critical component, to both Wennberg and the Foundation, was finding a way to get the information out to policy makers so that it would have a better chance of leading to change. It was again envisioned that this would be in a series of reports. The work evolved into what became known as *The Dartmouth Atlas of Health Care,* which was first published in 1996. "The *Atlas* was an afterthought, not the original thought, as the reports were," Wennberg said.

Schroeder had high hopes that the project would make the public and policy makers more aware of the differences in medical services throughout the nation, provide ammunition for efforts to improve quality of care, lead to less unnecessary care, and slow down the relentless climb of health care costs. "I expected Wennberg to create a resource others could use, especially people in communities where they could use the information to help make changes that were needed," Schroeder said. "Additionally, I thought it was a powerful tool to argue that cost containment does not mean lower quality."

The Foundation has supported what later became known as the Dartmouth Atlas Project with varying degrees of funding for the purchase of the Medicare database, the analysis by the working group at the Dartmouth-based Center for the Evaluative Clinical Sciences, which Wennberg directs, and the production of research reports. The Foundation's funding also covered the redesign of the *Atlas* Web site and the hiring of a communications specialist. In the 2004 round of grant making, the Foundation insisted that financial partners from health plans be sought to help cover the cost of purchasing and analyzing the claims database. This was meant to nudge the Dartmouth Atlas Project toward sustainability and to involve health plans more actively. The health plans that joined in, contributing from $100,000 to $250,000 annually each from their philanthropic arms, were WellPoint, United Healthcare, and Aetna. The California HealthCare Foundation also contributed.

—ᴟᴟ— The Dartmouth Atlas

Although *The Dartmouth Atlas of Health Care* was first envisioned as a series of state-by-state written reports on variations in the use of medical resources, it ultimately became a series of books that presented the data in a colorful way along with explanatory text. This was not intended to be a series of dreary medical journal articles with dry rundowns of multivariate analysis. With help from a member of the *Atlas* working group with expertise in mapping and a local firm talented at presenting information visually, what was unveiled after three years of research was a big $350 book with boldly shaded areas in various colors illustrating variations in care in a readily understood format. It was as though you could fly birdlike over the nation and see some locations that had, say, far more back surgeries or far fewer mastectomies than others. The *Atlas* measured resources such as hospitals, beds, and the supply of doctors and nurses, as well as Medicare spending, age-adjusted rates of surgery for every thousand Medicare enrollees in each hospital referral region, and much more. "The intention was always to have practical applications," Wennberg said in his cramped warren of offices at the Center for the Evaluative Clinical Sciences where he oversees the *Atlas,* an educational program, and other related endeavors.

Two more volumes of the *Atlas,* published in 1998 and 1999, explored end-of-life care, disparity in care, and quality of care measures— all areas of particular interest for the Robert Wood Johnson Foundation. The group would ultimately publish three state editions, nine regional editions, and three specialty care editions before the *Atlas* became exclusively a Web publication.

With a staff of about twenty economists, epidemiologists, statisticians, and other specialists putting it together, the *Atlas* has turned up numerous interesting facts. The cities of White Plains, New York, and San Francisco boast the most psychiatrists per capita, for example, and Boston, New York, Chicago, and Houston have the most physicians per capita. One statistic stands out above all others: medical spending is more than twice as high in some communities as it is in others—and not because people there are sicker or older. Particularly striking was a comparison between the $3,341 Medicare spent on each Minneapolis enrollee and the $8,414 it expended on each Miamian in 1996. Medicare recipients simply received more services and saw more doctors in Miami, which has become something of the poster child for the woes of too much hospitalization, diagnostic testing, specialist referrals, and office visits. The *Atlas* also found wide variation in mastectomies compared with lumpectomies for treatment of breast cancer and angioplasty versus bypass surgery to treat heart disease. In Birmingham, Alabama, for example, 7.7 per 1,000 Medicare recipients had bypass surgery, compared with 2.7 per 1,000 recipients in Albuquerque.

"It's data that tells you something about the world," said Megan McAndrew, editor of the *Atlas*. "The desirable thing would be that a doctor tells me I need back surgery, and I go to look it up. Am I in a place where every third person is getting back surgery? Should I go to Rochester, Minnesota, home of the legendary Mayo Clinic, which is known to be at the low end of the care spectrum with high quality, and see what they say?"

The *Atlas* made a strong nationwide case for what had been observed only in regions before: the kind of health care you receive depends on where you live rather than what is wrong with you. Furthermore, an examination of the death rates in low-use and high-use areas showed that people weren't dying sooner in areas where less care was being given.

In its exploration of end-of-life care, the *Atlas* showed that depending on where a patient lived, there were enormous differences in the chance of dying in a hospital bed or in the amount of time spent in the intensive care unit. Death in a hospital bed was, for example, most likely in New

Jersey, New York, southern California, and Miami. And the number of specialists seen, diagnostic tests, and office visits in high-use areas soared in the last six months of life when compared to low-use areas.

The *Atlas* also zeroed in on how well different locations were performing on quality indicators such as giving people older than sixty-five flu shots and checking lipid levels of people with diabetes. High-use and low-use areas alike fell short on these indicators. However, Rochester, Minnesota, boasted both low use of medical services and a high rate on quality measures.

In Michigan, the working group looked at private insurance data from Blue Cross Blue Shield of Michigan and found the same kinds of low-use and high-use patterns of health care services for patients with chronic health conditions. "The relationship between Medicare variations and variations for Blue Cross were the same," Wennberg said. This was important to document because it is virtually impossible to analyze variations in the private insurance market across the entire nation. "You can't get the data for the whole country," Wennberg said. "Private insurance is broken into hundreds of different companies and systems with their own data bases."

In 2000, the *Atlas* became a free Web-based publication as a way to lower costs and make the data accessible much faster than book publishing allows. The Dartmouth Atlas Project Web site posts topic papers, data quality measures, data sets, and downloads of previous editions of the book-form of the *Atlas* and is moving toward becoming more interactive. With the site's data, users can make their own tables and graphs comparing various hospitals or regions on a range of variables—just as the *Atlas* books did. With funding from the Robert Wood Johnson Foundation, the Web site is being remodeled to become even simpler and more useful. It will take fewer clicks to produce graphic displays of, say, the heart surgery rate for your region compared to the rest of the country. "We want to get this into a form that would enable your eighty-two-year-old father in Miami with prostate cancer to look up whether people are getting different answers in Fort Myers," McAndrew said.

In 2005, the Dartmouth Atlas Project moved in a new direction—one that it hoped would bring the case for corralling variation closer to home. Data pinpointed how individual California hospitals and hospital chains were performing and how they compared with each other from 1999 through 2003. This first hospital-specific data showed that the numbers of doctor visits and hospitalizations for chronically ill Medicare patients in Los Angeles were far higher than anywhere else in the state. Medicare spent $43,500 on hospitalized patients in the last two years of life in Los Angeles, the fifth-highest regional tab in the country. In contrast, it spent 20 percent less on patients in San Francisco, 36 percent less in San Diego, and 67 percent less in Sacramento. The *Atlas* provided detailed data on individual hospitals as well. For example, within the Los Angeles region, Medicare spent the most for hospitalizations and doctors at Garfield Medical Center in Monterey Park and the least at Foothill Presbyterian Hospital in Glendora. This kind of information, Wennberg states in a report, might be used to "stimulate major employers and payers to use data to direct their chronic disease populations away from high cost, high utilization hospitals to those that spend less and use less resources."[7] The financial benefits could be substantial. Consider this: Medicare could have saved $1.7 billion if Los Angeles's spending per person had been the same as Sacramento's, he wrote. The project planned to release the same kind of information for hospitals throughout the country in 2006.

—ⱴ— The Dartmouth Atlas and the Quality of Medical Care

"The existence of variation raises a number of important issues," the introduction to the first *Atlas* stated. "Foremost is the question 'Which rate is right?' Which pattern of resource allocation, and which pattern of utilization, is 'correct?'" Although Wennberg has speculated from the data that patients in high-use areas fare no better, an important related question also needed to be answered: If more health care isn't better care, could it possibly be worse?

Elliott Fisher, a Dartmouth Medical School professor and the co-principal investigator of the *Atlas,* set out to find the answer. Fisher submitted a grant request for the study to the Robert Wood Johnson

Foundation, which awarded it in 1997. (Funding also came from the National Institute on Aging and the National Cancer Institute.)

In a highly noted study published in the *Annals of Internal Medicine* in 2003, Fisher and his colleagues looked at the costs and health results of end-of-life care for people with hip fractures, colorectal cancer, or acute myocardial infarctions.[8] He found patients in the study's highest-spending areas got approximately 60 percent more health care—for minor procedures, physician visits, tests, and hospital and specialist use—but experienced no better health outcomes, satisfaction with their care, or superior functioning as a result. In fact, the extra care increased mortality by 2 to 5 percent—probably from patients' being subjected to the dangers inherent in being hospitalized such as increased risk of infection, Wennberg, Fisher, and others have theorized. The authors pointed out that if spending everywhere could be safely brought to the level of the low-use regions, Medicare spending would decline up to 30 percent annually—an enormous savings. "You know, it could have been that more was better—people in the higher spending areas could be getting all this care because they're sicker, Fisher said. "Or maybe they are benefiting from more health care. Now, as the result of our study, on the cross-sectional level, no one is arguing this is true anymore."

—⟋⟍— Factors Driving Health Care Spending

In 2002, Wennberg, Fisher, and Jonathan Skinner, a Dartmouth professor of economics and community and family medicine, laid out an analysis of the kinds of care that have a bearing on both quality and efficiency. In a paper of far-reaching impact funded by the National Institute on Aging and the Robert Wood Johnson Foundation, they divided health care services into three categories: effective care, preference-sensitive care, and supply-sensitive care. [9]

Effective care, the authors explained, is what people often mean by quality. These are the diagnostic tests and treatments that are accepted as standards of practice based on clinical trials or cohort studies, peer-reviewed articles, and general agreement. It is what people mean by evidence-based medicine, and is the minimum in quality care that all patients should expect from their health plans. Examples of effective care include a mammogram for breast cancer screening, tests for colon cancer, eye exams and HgA1c blood tests for diabetics, and prescribing aspirin and beta blockers for heart attack patients. The authors used Health Plan Employer Data and Information Set, or HEDIS, measures as indicators for effective medical care.

Unfortunately, the authors say, effective care services are underused all over the nation—and, surprisingly, patients in higher-spending Medicare regions underuse them just as much as those in lower-spending ones. Among the wide disparities in use of proven effective care that were cited: 5 to 92 percent of heart attack patients across the nation who would be ideal candidates for beta blockers actually received them; and the percentage of women between the ages of sixty-five and sixty-nine who had a mammogram once in a two-year period, the standard recommended by the United States Preventive Services Task Force, ranged between 21 and 77 percent.

Why aren't doctors following the evidence-based standards for medical practice and ensuring that their patients get immunizations, routine screenings, and treatments? The authors suggest that most doctors lack a system to track who needs them and then to get in touch with those patients.

Preference-sensitive care occurs when there is more than one treatment option for a health problem, with varying risks, benefits, and trade-offs to weigh. Patients in these situations need to acquire information to help them make a choice based on the best clinical evidence. However, the authors found, local medical opinion seems to be the determining factor most often. They pointed out that cardiac bypass surgery rates varied up to four times, from three per thousand in Albuquerque, New Mexico, to more than eleven per thousand in Redding, California. "The rates are strongly correlated with the numbers of per capita cardiac catheterization labs in the regions but not with illness rates as measured by the incidence of heart attacks in the region," they wrote. In other words, people get more bypass surgery in areas where there are more doctors and hospitals set up to treat heart attacks, not in areas where more people had heart attacks.

Decision-making is often difficult when there is scant medical literature about a condition. Patients suffering from lower back pain, for example, don't have clinical trials to look to for guidance on treatment alternatives. "It seems likely that individual physicians' opinions, rather than patients' preferences, explain the more than sixfold variation in surgery rates" found across the nation for lower back pain, the authors wrote. Moreover, the patterns for use of these preference-sensitive elective surgeries vary in idiosyncratic ways across the country, with a particular region being high in one type of surgery and low in another.

The best way to reduce unnecessary preference-sensitive care would be to inform patients of the various treatment options for their conditions so they can base a decision on their own values and preferences, the authors wrote. Shared decision-making, which Wennberg would always champion, can help patients understand their choices. Essential to this approach is a continued effort to expand the evidence base of medicine.

But the lion's share of excess medical care, where the stakes are the highest for finding a solution, was in what Wennberg, Fisher, and Skinner called supply-sensitive care, primarily for people with chronic diseases. More than 20 percent of what Medicare spends each year is on care for people who are in the last six months of their lives. The authors found that 41 percent of the wide variations in hospitalization, office visits, and diagnostic testing is determined by the local supply of specialists and hospital capacity. Doctors can find little guidance in medical texts and journals about how often to see chronically ill patients, when to hospitalize them, or when diagnostic tests should be ordered for them. Mostly, doctors are on their own, and the result is that end-of-life treatment is all over the map. For example, in Ogden, Utah, end-of-life patients were hospitalized an average of 4.6 days, while those in Newark, New Jersey, stayed in the hospital an average of 21.4 days.

The authors quantify the savings if high-spending areas were to receive the same amount of care as the low-spending areas: $40 billion in 1996 alone. They argued that although reducing disparities in this way would certainly upset many who would believe services were being taken away from them, patients would lose care of "little, or possibly negative, value." But simply putting a cap on services for each region is too simplistic and wouldn't tackle the bigger problem of improving the quality of care for Medicare patients. The authors' prescription for remedying Medicare's quality and efficiency problems includes improving systems to make sure effective care is given, expanding the knowledge base of medicine, developing a shared decision-making process, and having doctors practice medicine more conservatively.

—ᴍ— Variations in Care between Blacks and Whites and among Academic Medical Centers

Two other areas of study supported by the Foundation concerned health care disparities between African Americans and whites, and whether pronounced variation exists in the best of American hospitals, its academic medical centers.

In 2003, an Institute of Medicine study, *Unequal Treatment: Confronting the Racial and Ethnic Disparities in Health Care,* found marked disparities in the health care treatment and outcomes of black patients, especially for heart disease.[10] Probing further, in a 2005 study, Jonathan Skinner and his co-authors found that heart attack patients admitted to hospitals that care for a disproportionate number of African Americans stood an 18 percent higher chance of dying within three months than if they had gone to a hospital that serves disproportionately white patients.[11] "We're saying a very important source of the disparity is what hospital you go to, at least in relation to thirty-day survival rates after a heart attack," Skinner said in an interview. "All the disparity is because black people went to different hospitals than whites. We're not talking about disparity or treatment within hospitals." Skinner described this as a "neglected form of discrimination" much akin to how school segregation led to lesser schools for black students.

Another study reported that the kind of variation found generally throughout the country even occurs at the seventy-seven hospitals *U.S. News & World Report* anointed the nation's "best" for 2001. This study found "extensive variation" in end-of-life care among these highly respected hospitals. The difference was attributed to the availability of more hospital beds and physicians per capita.[12]

─ᴠᴠ─ The Practical Application of the Dartmouth Atlas

By 2006, Wennberg had become something of a legend. He is invariably described as indefatigable, stubborn, brilliant, and fearless. He brought us the counterintuitive conclusion that more health care can be worse health care. He has waged a lifelong campaign of making people aware of the variations in health care occurring in town after town. Today he is considered a towering figure, his work regarded as seminal and an underpinning of the movement to improve the quality of health care, base medicine on solid proof of what works, and bring patients into the decision-making loop about their own medical care. "His work is the most important health services work of his generation," said the Institute for Healthcare Improvement's Donald Berwick, the institute's president and chief executive officer and himself a pillar in the ongoing quality quest. "He was the guy who first started to turn the lights on variation, which was not a popular inquiry when he started . . . He has shown the chaos of medical care that is not committed to evidence."

So powerful is the basic message of the *Dartmouth Atlas* that it has become part of the DNA of those in health policy and services today. As it has evolved, the *Atlas* has been recognized as providing superb data and analyses and as an asset to the medical field. Few people quibble any longer with the basic contention that there are huge, nonsensical variations in office visits to doctors and specialists, surgeries, hospital stays, lab tests, and the like, and that they represent a mammoth amount of waste. "What Wennberg has done with the *Atlas* is extraordinarily important," said physician Robert Brook, a corporate fellow at RAND and director of RAND's Health Sciences Program, who himself is a prominent leader in the movement to improve the quality of care. "He called our attention, when nobody wanted to do it, to the notion that you need to look at what things are being done on a geographic basis, controlling for age, sex, and race. There are huge differences. Something there is wrong."

Jack Hadley, a principal research associate at the Urban Institute, also offers high praise. "The *Atlas* has been very influential and persuasive mainly because it's very easy to understand most of what they found," he said. "The variations and amount of spending per Medicare beneficiary across the country appear to be much larger than any variation in health. They've been hammering away at this theme over and over. It seems to consistently find the same results. That has added to its persuasiveness."

But Brook, Hadley, and others do have substantive bones to pick as well. While Wennberg asserts that decreasing the supply of care in the high-intensity areas would be beneficial, Brook and his colleagues have conducted studies showing that the level of use of a medical service does not correlate to whether it's appropriate.[13] "Simply cutting supply therefore would cut out things that are both needed and unneeded and we ought to be able to do better than that," Brook said. He advocates coupling the geographic disparity data with a look at the clinical appropriateness of the care that is either going to be or has been delivered. This means stepping into the clinical environment or going back and reading patients' charts. By reviewing the clinical evidence for a procedure and the physician's judgment, as Brook and his colleagues have done, one can tell whether the health benefit of performing that procedure exceeds the health risk—and determine whether care was appropriate and thus warranted. In his own work with colleagues, Brook found that the same proportion of people get care they need and don't need in both high-use and low-use areas. "The net impact is very little impact on health."

Hadley, too, believes that Wennberg and the *Atlas* have not definitively answered what causes the variations, and says he's unconvinced that their theories will prove correct. With some *Atlas* hospital referral areas far larger than others, Hadley wonders if much of the individual variation is being lumped all together—some patients getting much more care and some very little within the hospital referral areas—and thus distorting the average.

"To say that nobody should spend more than what is spent in the median area could mean very dramatic changes for individuals who would in fact benefit from more care," said David Cutler, a Harvard University health economist. Cutler observes that Wennberg's work doesn't take into account the last thirty years of remarkable medical advances that have improved survival rates for many serious conditions, such as heart disease and cancer. To him, too much care is just fine.

Wennberg's footprints can be detected in a number of policy areas. He advocated for a federal agency that would fund outcomes research to increase the evidence base for medicine, which resulted in the establishment of the Agency for Health Care Policy and Research, now called the Agency for Healthcare Research and Quality, or AHRQ, in 1989. He pushed for the Patient Outcomes Research Teams that during the 1990s recommended how to treat patients with common high-risk and costly health conditions for which options weren't clear. Although AHRQ does less of this kind of research now, other federal agencies such as the National Institutes of Health have picked up some of it. His inspiration can also be seen in pay-for-performance experiments, both in government and some private insurance plans, that reward doctors for using quality measures and providing fewer services.

Yet a nagging doubt remains. Why hasn't the *Atlas* had more impact? While some health plans, such as Intermountain Healthcare, a Salt Lake City–based managed care system, are beginning to use the *Atlas*'s data to reduce their own variations, the *Atlas* has been far less influential in the real world of health care than its supporters expected it to be. This raises the question: After so many years of showing ever more precisely just how much unwarranted variation and wasteful care is being given to Medicare patients, why do the same patterns of disparity persist year after year?

To most observers, it is a matter of politics, entrenched interests, and the complexity of changing the status quo. "If you're a congressman, what should you do about this?" David Cutler asked. "It's all about when there are too many doctors and hospitals, bad things happen. What do you do about that? Close hospitals? Restrict the numbers of doctors that can practice in South Florida? And how do you do that—issue something like taxi medallions for them?"

David Durenberger, the former Republican senator from Minnesota and a health policy expert, said that if the *Atlas* data had been as developed as it is today back in the 1980s, when several dozen senators and representatives were making changes to Medicare policy, it could have provided direction and answers. But the time has not been right in the early 2000s for national political leaders to take on variations in spending on chronic illness and care in the last two years of life. "The problem is not that the data is obscure but that the leadership is not there in Congress," Durenberger said. "What preoccupies the politicians is the elections."

Margaret O'Kane, president of the National Committee for Quality Assurance, has spent considerable time with Wennberg on Capitol Hill as he has urged elected representatives to recognize the disparities in health care services in the nation and make changes in Medicare. "The notion of shifting medical spending so that high-use areas are put on a 'diet' is a nonstarter in Congress, where lobbyists for hospitals and physician organizations are highly influential," she said. "I can't imagine that happening unless there were an extremely powerful constituency pushing for it."

According to O'Kane, the Dartmouth Atlas Project should look beyond preparing its good "wonky" papers for medical and health policy research journals. "They need to use a different communications strategy," she said. "It needs to be a broader campaign—in the business press where employers will read about it and say, 'Why are we putting up with this?' I think a lot of large corporations don't know about this. If they read about it in *Fortune* or *Business Week,* they'll pay more attention. The business press is an unexploited opportunity."

The Urban Institute's Jack Hadley summed up what the program has accomplished. "Wennberg's impact is not so much in policies implemented but in raising very key questions that policy makers are now trying to better understand and potentially use to make policy changes," he said.

—⁓— Conclusion

Despite these concerns, there is little doubt of the influence of Wennberg and the *Dartmouth Atlas* in health policy circles. "He has very patiently and thoroughly dealt with all of the 'yes, buts,' and what he's got is a set of findings that are too large in size and carefully done to brush off," said Henry Aaron, a senior fellow in economic studies with the Brookings Institution.

Not only that, Wennberg has built an outstanding team of health services researchers at the Center for the Evaluative Clinical Sciences. Researchers such as Elliott Fisher and Jonathan Skinner are already highly regarded in their own right and have branched out in important new directions.

After all these years, Wennberg, who says he won't retire until "the variations go away," is philosophical about the prospects of seeing that happening. "It depends on whether you're viewing the glass as nine-tenths empty or one-tenth full," he told the *Wall Street Journal* in 2002.[14] "Changing the health care system is like changing the Catholic Church. It takes a long time."

Notes

1. Wennberg, J. E., Fisher, E. S., and Skinner, J. S. "Geography and the Debate over Medicare Reform." *Health Affairs,* Web Exclusive, February 13, 2002, w96–w114.
2. Wennberg, J. E., and Gittelsohn, A. "Small Area Variations in Health Care Delivery." *Science,* 1973, *182,* 1102–1108.
3. For Maine: See Wennberg, J. E., and Gittelsohn, A. "Health Care Delivery in Maine I: Patterns of Use of Common Surgical Procedures." *The Journal of the Maine Medical Association,* 1975, *66*(5), 123–149.
   For New England: See Wennberg, J. E., and Gittelsohn, A. "Variations in Medical Care Among Small Areas." *Scientific American,* 1982, *246*(4), 120–134.
4. Wennberg, J. E. and Gittelsohn, A. "Variations in Medical Care Among Small Areas." *Scientific American,* 1982, *246*(4), 120–134.
5. Wennberg, J. E., Freeman, J. L., and Culp, W. J. "Are Hospital Services Rationed in New Haven or Over-Utilised in Boston?" *Lancet,* 1987, *1*(8543), 1185–1189.
6. Fisher, E. S., Wennberg, D. E., Stukel, T. A., Gottlieb, D., Lucas, F. L., and Pinder, E. L. "The Implications of Regional Variations in Medicare Spending. Part 2: Health Outcomes and Satisfaction with Care." *Annals of Internal Medicine,* 2003, *138*(4), 288–298.
7. Wennberg, J. E., Fisher, E. S., Baker, L., Sharp, S. M., and Bronner, K. K. "Evaluating the Efficiency of California Providers in Caring for Patients with Chronic Illness." *Health Affairs,* Web Exclusive, November 16, 2005, *24*(6), w5-526–w5-543. Quote from page w5-541.

8. Fisher, E. S., Wennberg, J. E., Stukel, T. A., Gottlieb, Daniel J., Lucas, F. L., and Pinder, E. "The Implications of Regional Variations in Medicare Spending. Part 1: The Content, Quality, and Accessibility of Care." *Annals of Internal Medicine,* 2003, *138*(4), 273–288.

   And see Fisher, E. S., Wennberg, J. E., Stukel, T. A., Gottlieb, D. J., Lucas, F. L., and Pinder, E. "The Implications of Regional Variations in Medicare Spending. Part 2: Health Outcomes and Satisfaction with Care." *Annals of Internal Medicine,* 2003, *138*(4), 288–298.

9. Wennberg, J. E., Fisher, E. S., and Skinner, J. S. "Geography and the Debate over Medicare Reform." *Health Affairs,* Web Exclusive, February 13, 2002, w96–w114.

10. Smedley, B. D., Stith, A. Y., and Nelson, A. R. (eds.) Institute of Medicine Committee on Understanding and Eliminating Racial and Ethnic Disparities in Health Care, *Unequal Treatment: Confronting the Racial and Ethnic Disparities in Health Care.* Washington, D.C.: The National Academies Press, 2003.

11. Skinner, J. S., Chandra, A., Staiger, D., Lee, J., McClellan, M. "Mortality After Acute Myocardial Infarction in Hospitals that Disproportionately Treat African-Americans." *Circulation,* 2005, *112*(17), 2634–2641.

12. Wennberg, J. E., Fisher, E. S., Stukel, T. A., Skinner, J. S., Sharp, S. M., and Bronner, K. K. "Use of Hospitals, Physician Visits, and Hospice Care During the Last Six Months of Life Among Cohorts Loyal to Highly Respected Hospitals in the United States." *British Medical Journal,* 2004, *328,* 607–610.

13. Chassin, M. R., Kosecoff, J., Park, R. E., Winslow, C. M., Kahn, K. L., Merritt, N., Keesey, J., Fink, A., Solomon, D., and Brook, R. H. "Does Inappropriate Use Explain Geographic Variations in the Use of Health Care Services? A Study of Three Procedures." *Journal of the American Medical Association,* 1987, *258*(8), 2533–2537.

14. Wessel, D. "The Medical Mystery of Sun City and Other Health-Care Oddities." *The Wall Street Journal,* March 21, 2003.

3

Improving Chronic Illness Care

Irene M. Wielawski

Editors' Introduction

One of the Robert Wood Johnson Foundation's priorities is improving the quality of care delivered to people with chronic illnesses. Improving quality of care was one of the three priorities approved by the board in 1972, shortly after the Foundation became a national philanthropy, and it has been a Foundation concern ever since. Among its other efforts, the Foundation has supported quality-measurement standards developed by the National Committee for Quality Assurance, commissioned major studies on quality of care by the Institute of Medicine, and funded *The Dartmouth Atlas of Health Care*, which is the subject of the previous chapter in this *Anthology*.

In this chapter, freelance journalist Irene Wielawski, a frequent contributor to the *Anthology* series, explores a Foundation-supported initiative called Improving Chronic Illness Care, a pioneering effort spearheaded by Dr. Edward Wagner of the Group Health Cooperative in Seattle to provide medical care for chronically ill people, whatever their condition. In tracing the history of the Foundation's efforts to improve quality of care, Wielawski concludes that many of the foundation's past efforts focused on specific illnesses such as asthma, diabetes, or depression. In contrast, the chronic care model developed by Wagner, around which the Improving Chronic Illness Care Program was built, applies to a broad range of chronic illnesses and serves as a roadmap for physicians to organize their practices to meet the often complex needs of chronically ill people.

In fact, the chronic care model calls for a structural change in the way people with illnesses are cared for, and the participation of nurses, social workers, and patients themselves. This chapter highlights how difficult it is to change what goes on in physicians' offices and to modify practices that have been entrenched for many years. The challenge is now one of moving an apparently effective way of improving quality from an experiment carried out primarily in health maintenance organizations to the mainstream of health care practice.

To hear Carolee Ross tell it, she had to come to "Podunk" to get a proper diagnosis for symptoms that she had experienced for several years: persistent thirst, frequent urination, ravenous hunger, and a shaky, sweaty feeling that would come over her without warning. These are classic symptoms of diabetes, an illness that runs in Ross's family. But in all the years that she had been complaining, none of her doctors in an affluent suburb of New York City did a thorough workup.

What Ross considers Podunk is a rural section of southern Rhode Island known as Chariho, for the three towns—Charlestown, Richmond, and Hopkinton—that send children to the regional high school. Ross landed there in 2002 after she and her husband were downsized out of their corporate jobs. By selling their pricey home and relocating to a place like Chariho, Ross figured that they could buy a nice house, start a home-based business, and still have money left over for expenses. It didn't work out that way. Health insurance remained out of reach, forcing a reluctant Ross to seek care at the local sliding fee scale clinic, Wood River Health Services.

"I never thought I'd find myself in that kind of place," says Ross, who had prided herself on going to only the best private doctors. But what seemed like a huge comedown turned out to be a stroke of luck.

The physician's assistant who conducted the new patient interview immediately flagged Ross as a possible diabetic. He then ushered her into tests that confirmed it, which brought the clinic's diabetes team into play. The comprehensive education and treatment plan they devised quite literally changed Ross's life, helping her confront lifestyle excesses that were ruining her health—as well as prejudices about medical care quality that she had brought from her past life.

"I had a wonderful, caring relationship with my doctor, but I'm sorry to say she never took my diabetes symptoms seriously," Ross says. "All she did was a simple urine test, and when it came back negative, she suggested stress might be the explanation—as if this was all in my head!"

That Ross was diagnosed so quickly at Wood River is no accident. The health center and the state of Rhode Island are among several dozen loosely aggregated collaborative projects in a national experiment called Improving Chronic Illness Care, or ICIC. In 1998, the Robert Wood Johnson Foundation authorized $25 million over five years for ICIC. The program's purpose was to address one of the standout areas of illogic in American health care—the treatment of patients with ongoing but incurable illness.

The idea behind ICIC is to marry medical science with redesigned health care delivery systems so chronic patients in any setting—clinic, hospital, physician's office, or health maintenance organization—can receive prompt diagnoses and care that helps them avoid debilitating and expensive complications. The logic is powerful, backed by research and demographic trends foreshadowing more chronic patients as the baby boom generation ages. A "no-brainer" is how national proponents like to sum it up.

But the grantees who took up ICIC's challenge to reengineer their health care organizations aren't so breezy. Indeed, their descriptions of what it has taken to upend health care business as usual sound more like the rhetoric of the Prussian military strategist Carl von Clausewitz than modern health reform theory. Among the obstacles they cite are a century of clinical and cultural maxims about the role of physicians, extreme fragmentation of purpose and incentives in American health care, and a payment system that runs in the opposite direction.

—ᴡ— A Fragmented Approach to Treating Chronic Illness

Like Ross's former doctor, the health care system is geared to hard evidence of medical need. That's great if you've been pulled broken and bloody from a car wreck, but not so great if you're in the early stages of diabetes or asthma or heart disease. Though similarly life threatening, these illnesses erode health over years, not minutes. Symptoms may be subtle, delaying diagnosis by busy clinicians. Treatment is often laborious; chronic conditions can complicate even the most routine of medical procedures. And there's little reward for conscientious clinicians because the so-called "acute" care bias in the health care system extends to its payment formulas. Simply put, doctors and hospitals make more money amputating the gangrenous limbs of poorly controlled diabetics, performing bypass surgery on patients with advanced heart disease and hospitalizing asthmatics than they do helping these patients avoid such acute exacerbations of underlying illness.

The acute care bias persists despite scientific evidence that early diagnosis and management of specific chronic conditions not only is good for patients but also has the potential to significantly restrain growth in the nation's health care bill—now $1.9 trillion,[1] or 16 percent of the gross domestic product—by reducing hospitalization and other costly measures. The math here is complicated and quite theoretical, since there has been no long-term test of researchers' projections across the full spectrum of chronic illness. Demographics, however, add force to their arguments for improving the care of people like Carolee Ross. An estimated total of 133 million people in the United States— nearly half of all Americans—have at least one chronic condition, and that number is expected to swell to 171 million by 2030 as a result of the aging of the population. Moreover, researchers believe that these projections understate the potential demand on disease management services. It is estimated that nearly one third of the people suffering from diabetes alone remain undiagnosed.[2]

Health care leaders have long been aware of this trajectory. Chronic illness has displaced the nineteenth-century acute threats that spawned our health care system: contagious disease, farm accidents, blade and bullet mishaps, and so on. People a hundred years ago simply didn't survive cancers, flaws in metabolism, or failing organs. The twentieth century brought rapid progress in medical science—the development of antibiotics and life-sustaining drugs such as insulin, surgical interventions, and a host of new technologies that made it possible for the chronically ill to live longer. The new challenge was to minimize the disruption of illness at home and at work.

At the Robert Wood Johnson Foundation, ICIC was preceded by two decades of programs to invent or refine services for patients in need of extra help. The Foundation categorized them as "special populations," including the elderly, children, people with physical or mental handicaps, and those with chronic illness. Among the chronic illness initiatives were several that experimented with new approaches to specific diseases such as AIDS or asthma. Others took aim at systemic gaps, and sought to augment support for people with long-term illness. A particular need was for help in day-to-day medical management. Physicians and other clinicians sometimes were too rushed to discuss diet, exercise, or self-care techniques, and their offices weren't organized to connect patients with services in the larger community.

To address these deficiencies, the Foundation funded experiments in case management and patient education, as well as integrated social and health services needed by complex patients. The Chronic Disease Care Program (1979–84) used nurse managers to organize consultations and other services for severely ill patients, and also teach them how to care for themselves. The goal was to reduce hospitalizations and institutionalization, but it proved to be an uphill battle because doctors and administrators weren't part of the program and didn't always back the nurses. The Program for the Health-Impaired Elderly (1980–85) moved case management work out of the medical office and into community organizations that also saw to transportation, meals, and other needs of geriatric patients. The Chronic Mental Illness Program (1985–1992) worked similarly on behalf of people with psychiatric illness, helping them to navigate the maze of existing federal, state, and local programs, all with different funding streams and eligibility criteria. The Health Care for the Homeless Program (1983–1990) targeted people living on the streets and in shelters. But the homeless program emphasized primary medical care. Mental health problems, although rampant in this population, were not addressed.[3]

A number of initiatives targeted social needs of fragile or medically impaired populations. The Supportive Services Program in Senior Housing (1987–1995) sought to build capacity for services beyond the standard landlord-tenant relationship so that, for an additional fee, elderly residents could receive help with housekeeping, repairs, and miscellaneous chores. The Program on Dementia Care and Respite Services (1987–1992) promoted adult day care centers for severely demented persons still living with their families.

What stands out from a review of these programs is how scattershot they were, addressing the isolated needs of people with particular handicaps but offering no systematic solution for patients, families, health care facilities, and clinicians to collectively meet the challenges posed by chronic conditions. There also was little effort to utilize lessons across programs. After all, if residents in senior housing need help with chores and repairs, it's likely that people with health or mobility problems do, too. It wouldn't be stretching it to describe the Foundation's early chronic illness portfolio as an "acute care" approach to the symptoms of health system failure that ignored the underlying disease—an antiquated structure that divides patients by diagnosis and circumstance instead of comprehensively addressing chronic patients' needs. Anne Weiss, the senior program officer who heads the Foundation's quality team, characterizes these earlier initiatives as a form of "parallel play," borrowing a phrase used by developmental psychologists to describe toddlers playing side by side but with no apparent interaction. The Foundation's chronic illness initiatives of the 1980s and early 1990s, she says, "had general common ground, but some were systems-oriented and some were patient education-oriented and some had a different focus altogether."

This piecemeal approach was mirrored nationally as scholars, institutions, advocacy groups, and government agencies sought variously to address weaknesses in health care quality and delivery but stopped short of solutions that could be applied to all chronic conditions. At Dartmouth Medical School, John Wennberg pioneered the study of regional variation in medical practice, showing, for example, differences in the rates of specific medical procedures such as coronary artery bypass surgery and hysterectomy that lacked scientific rationale. Donald Berwick, at the Institute for Healthcare Improvement, focused on medical errors and strategies to improve patient care safety. Federal and state officials explored ways to tweak reimbursement formulas in order to encourage better care of chronically ill patients covered by Medicare and Medicaid.

Finally, there was the broad public education effort that accompanied managed care to convert sick people into informed consumers of health care services.

While each of these efforts attempted to improve the quality of medical care, they lacked a coordinated action plan that would meld the interests of patients and their families in obtaining good care with those of hospitals and clinicians juggling twin mandates to practice good medicine *and* make a living under restrictive payment formulas.

—ᄴ— The Chronic Care Model

Could such a plan be devised and implemented within the existing structures of health care in the United States? This was the question posed by the Foundation in the early 1990s to Edward Wagner, an internist and director of the Seattle-based MacColl Institute for Healthcare Innovation at the Center for Health Studies, Group Health Cooperative. Wagner is a longtime proponent of chronic disease management to minimize acute illness. He first came to the Foundation's attention in 1992 as a grantee under the Chronic Care in HMOs program, during which time he identified specific shortcomings of primary care offices and organizational changes needed to enhance services for chronic patients.

Among the problems identified by Wagner:

- The typical primary care office is set up to respond to acute illness rather than to anticipate and respond proactively to patients' needs. Chronically ill patients, however, need the latter approach in order to avoid acute episodes of illness and debilitating complications.

- Chronically ill patients aren't sufficiently informed about their conditions, nor are they supported in self-care beyond the doctor's office. This lack has consequences beyond preventable exacerbations of illness. Children with poorly controlled asthma, for example, can end up permanently sidelined from sports, playground games, and other activities important to physical and social development.

- Physicians are too busy to educate and support chronically ill patients to the degree necessary to keep them healthy.

Wagner's solution is to replace the traditional physician-centric office structure with one that supports clinical teamwork in collaboration with the patient. The concept extends beyond the health care organization to collaborative relationships in the community—say, with the local YMCA's cardio-fitness program. Wagner called his design the "chronic care model." Under the model, physicians, nurses, case managers, dieticians, and patient educators collectively share responsibility for patients' well-being. They are supported in this mission by administrative staff and technology relevant to the task. For example, Wagner's model calls for investment in computerized patient records and special software to organize disease data and alert members of the care team to patients' needs.

The chronic care model defines six elements whose coordination is necessary for high-quality disease management:

- Community Resources. Doctors' offices and clinics should identify existing programs and encourage patients to participate.

- Health system. Health care organizations must make excellence a priority and pursue it visibly. Essential to achieving this is top management support and open communication on error and failings as well as strategies for improvement.

- Self-management support. Clinicians should set a tone of collaboration with chronic patients, and encourage their participation in setting goals and fine-tuning treatment.

- Delivery system design. To move from the one-on-one doctor/patient relationship to teamwork, the clinical staff needs defined roles and tasks. Follow-up with patients is essential so they feel supported in self-management efforts outside the medical office.

- Decision support. To link treatment to research evidence, clinicians must have explicit guidelines, whether the question is scientific (drug doses) or psychosocial (how best to motivate overweight diabetics to diet).

- Clinical information systems. Computers can efficiently deliver disease management information, including care guidelines, test results, and even pop-up reminders about individual patients. They also facilitate so-called population studies of, say, all diabetics in the office; the care team can measure their performance against quality benchmarks.

By integrating these elements into primary care practice, Wagner says, health care organizations are better able to stay on top of clinical responsibilities while helping patients become active participants in their care. The result is win-win all around, he says. Patients are healthier, providers are cheered and motivated by evidence of a job well done, and the health care system saves money.

—∿— The Improving Chronic Illness Care Program

Wagner's early trials of the chronic care model took place at Group Health Cooperative, a 590,000-member health maintenance organization based in Seattle. He chose to test it on diabetes, a long-term chronic illness with known complications related to poor disease management. Some 15,000 diabetics spread among 200 primary care providers in twenty-five affiliated clinics participated in the experiment. Over a five-year period, the percentage of these patients with up-to-date screenings for eye, foot, and other complications rose; blood sugar levels and the regularity of monitoring improved; patients reported higher satisfaction with their care; and the utilization of acute care services decreased. Specifically, Wagner and colleagues reported, inpatient admissions went down 17 percent for diabetic patients, and office visits also declined, for an overall cost savings of $62 per member per month.[4]

Tracy Orleans, a senior scientist/program officer and distinguished scholar at the Foundation who had previously worked on chronic disease management programs, said that she had "never seen more exciting work" than Wagner's. It coincided with growing disenchantment at the Foundation with its "let a thousand flowers bloom" approach to improving chronic illness and a search for something "more prescriptive," Orleans says. After funding the chronic care model's initial trial through the Chronic Care in HMOs program (1993–97), the Foundation offered Wagner additional grant support to refine the model. This work took place between 1994 and 1998. It included compiling best practices guidelines from the research on chronic illness management, and a conference of experts who provided valuable feedback on the model.

Wagner says this lead-up to ICIC was a period of great uncertainty. Would clinicians oriented to treating individual patients be receptive to systematizing disease management by diagnosis category, and even across chronic conditions? "Everything at the time was in disease silos," Wagner recalls. "Patient education was in a funny state because there was evidence that it wasn't working and that the field was floundering. There was a *Journal of Chronic Disease* that actually changed its name to *Journal of Clinical Epidemiology* to go along with the fashion of the time. In short, there was no field called chronic disease management." But Wagner says interest built as he and his team began to publish their ideas. Several organizations interested in health care quality and system reform eventually joined ICIC as collaborators, including the Institute for Healthcare Improvement, the Bureau of Primary Health Care of the U.S. Health Resources and Services Administration, the Joint Commission on Accreditation of Healthcare Organizations, and the National Committee for Quality Assurance.

The final design for ICIC included three major components:

- A grant program for research on system barriers to state-of-the-art chronic disease care. These included studies of how to integrate community resources into clinical practice, adapt disease management tools to small physician practices, use web-TV technology to teach self-management techniques to isolated rural patients, and enhance the flow of medical information as patients move from one health care setting to another.

■ Real-world tests of the chronic care model in a range of practice settings—private physicians' offices, government-subsidized clinics, hospital-based outpatient clinics, and other places where the chronically ill might go for medical care. To teach grantees how to re-engineer their work environments, ICIC teamed up with the Institute for Healthcare Improvement to run training programs called the Breakthrough Series. These included national meetings, group coaching, and feedback for clinical leadership teams designated by their health care organizations. Their assignment was to implement the chronic care model in their workplaces, but also to stay in touch with the other teams as part of an idea-sharing collaborative. As of January, 2006, more than 1,300 health care organizations had participated in ICIC collaboratives.

■ A technical assistance center to help others utilize the lessons of ICIC. The center maintains a public access website, www. improvingchroniccare.org, with links to current research, resources, and reports on the experiences of ICIC grantees.

While the chronic care model is certainly prescriptive, dictating criteria and processes for changing medical office design and practice, ICIC presented it as a flexible tool, designed for adaptation to the great variety of primary care settings in the United States. For example, grantees were encouraged to modify the recommended form for interviewing new patients. The only condition was that these modifications had to be scientifically tested to document better results—Carolee Ross, say, receiving a prompt diagnosis of diabetes after years of neglect.

This opened the door to innovation at every level of ICIC, creating the same dynamic collaboration between the national program office and its grantees that the chronic care model espoused for patients and the health care team. Grantees said they were energized by this freedom to tailor the model to their work environments. ICIC, in turn, disseminated grantee contributions in papers and via its website, enabling a three-physician practice in Montana, say, to learn from a similar operation in Rhode Island.

Among many lessons from the field was that such small practices lacked sufficient capital (for data collection and information systems) and staff (for patient education and support) to comprehensively implement the model. Partly in response to this, ICIC shifted its collaborative base from nationally scattered experimental sites to local, regional, and statewide collaboratives. The thinking, according to Wagner, was that collaboratives linked by geography and markets would have a better chance of influencing health insurers and government and private sector agencies to kick in up-front financial support on the evidence of cost savings down the road.

"Money isn't the problem; misdirected money is the problem," says Wagner, who estimates that for certain chronic illnesses, notably congestive heart failure, a $300 to $500 investment per patient per year yields health care system savings of up to $1,000.

─ᘘ─ The ICIC Battlefield

While no blood was shed during ICIC's experiments with the chronic care model, participants sometimes reached for warlike metaphors to convey how wrenching the process was for individuals and organizations to change longstanding ways of practicing medicine. The fact is that ICIC was as much an experiment in social change as a clinical trial, despite its emphasis on quantifying proof of better disease management. Patients didn't necessarily jump at the chance to become collaborators and self-managers after years of following doctors' orders. Nor were physicians immediately comfortable with transferring clinical responsibilities to colleagues traditionally viewed as subordinates. Michael Tronolone, medical director of the Polyclinic, a Seattle physicians' group and ICIC grantee, said the clinic's chronic care team sometimes had to resort to "guerilla warfare" to bring resistant physicians around. "It's really a tactical issue," he said. "You take on one physician at a time."

Pat Schultz, a nurse at Wood River Health Services in Rhode Island, where Carolee Ross learned that she had diabetes, says the chronic care model's emphasis on clinical teamwork explodes medicine's traditional hierarchy, forcing recognition of other health care professionals as equal or superior to physicians in certain patient care tasks.

"Years ago, it was always nurse is handmaiden to the doctor," Schultz says. "You did no more and no less than you were told. This requires us to put our titles and our hats aside to figure out how to make things better for patients, not easier for us as providers or better for us as a business."

Much has been published about ICIC's experience and clinical results, as well as the arduous process of changing entrenched but no longer useful ways of doing business. The experiences of selected patients and sites can serve to illuminate both the difficulties and the promise of improving chronic illness care. The accounts that follow all involve diabetes, predominantly type II, or adult-onset, diabetes, a widespread chronic illness that has typically afflicted middle-aged and older Americans but now is showing up in younger patients.

Roughly 21 million people, or 7 percent of the American population, suffer from type-2 diabetes, in which the body fails to utilize the hormone insulin or produce it in quantities sufficient to metabolize glucose—an important fuel for cells. People with Type II diabetes usually still produce insulin, which distinguishes them from the 5 percent to 10 percent of Americans with Type I, or juvenile, diabetes, who don't.[5] Neither type is curable, and both can lead to dangerously high levels of glucose in the blood. Left untreated, diabetes impairs kidneys, hearts, eyes, nerves, and circulation. Treatment includes synthetic insulin, diet, and exercise, as well as close monitoring for complications. Three-quarters of the ICIC grantees chose diabetes to roll out the chronic care model in their organizations, despite being offered three other chronic illnesses: asthma, congestive heart failure, and depression. Grantees cited its prevalence as one reason, but emphasized a second one in light of ICIC's mandate to measure clinical performance by scientific standards. Diabetes produces unusually hard data, compared to other chronic conditions. Because success can be documented, diabetes has more heft as a driver of system change than other illnesses where the science isn't so clear and the cost of failing to achieve clinical excellence cannot be so cleanly projected.

Patient: Donald W. Bangs

Donald Bangs was still teaching sixth grade at a Seattle middle school when he was diagnosed with Type II diabetes in 1980. "I'm 6 feet tall and I weighed about 212 pounds, but the weight was going off fast because I was sick and thirsty all the time," he says. "I told my sister because she had diabetes and our father and grandmother had it, so I knew a bit about the symptoms."

Still, Bangs didn't call his doctor right away. Instead, he waited several months, until it was time for his annual teacher's physical. Bangs' own hunch about diabetes was quickly confirmed. He left his doctor's office with a packet of literature about diet restrictions and other measures to control blood sugar—the standard patient education packet at the time. "It was so screwy that I couldn't eat this and I had to eat that," Bangs says, recalling his initial confusion over how to care for himself.

Over the years, Bangs' doctors at Seattle's Polyclinic added new regimens and medications, though still without much explanation. Bangs' need for synthetic formulations of the glucose-metabolizing hormone insulin steadily increased.

"You're always wondering when you've got something like this, 'Am I doing the right thing?' My sister had insulin reactions [from overdosing] all the time. Her sons are on the fire department, and the 911 call would come in and they'd say, 'That's mother.' They'd have to rush over there and feed her sugar and put that glucose needle in her arm. She died in 1999, but her last years were terrible. I went over to visit her one time at Swedish Hospital and it was bad—tubes in her all over the place."

By contrast, Bangs says he's never had an insulin reaction. He attributes this to having taught science, which made him curious about the physiology of diabetes and also a careful reader of informational pamphlets. But Bangs gives much credit to the Polyclinic, which began using the chronic care model in 2001 to manage diabetic patients, and stepped-up emphasis on patient education and self-management. Bangs, who injects himself with insulin four times a day, says he monitors the effects by pricking himself before and after meals to measure blood glucose concentrations. He records these on a chart provided by the Polyclinic, and also notes what and when he eats each day. He then plots the blood sugars scores on graph paper. Both chart and graph go with Bangs to every Polyclinic visit. The visits include eye, foot, blood pressure, and other screening tests, as well as HbA1c blood tests—a nationally recognized standard of diabetes control that measures blood glucose over time. Normal scores are 5 percent or less; diabetics are considered in good control if they score below 7.

"The numbers show that you really can help your health," says Bangs, whose HbA1c's have been as high as 12. Working with the Polyclinic's diabetes care team has been rewarding, primarily for reasons of health but also, says Bangs, because of the feeling of self-mastery he gets from success: "When my doctor told me one day that I got a 7.1, wow, I felt like I'd won the $100,000 lottery!"

Physician: Gregory John

Gregory John, a fifty-four-year-old internist, is a partner in the Seattle group practice where Donald Bangs is a patient. He was one of the first Polyclinic doctors to convert his practice to the chronic care model and embrace its systematic team approach to managing chronic illness. But John is quick to note that it was not love at first sight. On the contrary, John says he expected this latest health reform scheme to be little more than a paperwork exercise—time-consuming, for sure, but of little benefit to patients or his practice.

"I already had a very busy practice and I already had to go to a lot of meetings, so I was very resistant to doing all the work involved in learning these new ways to take care of people," says John, who nevertheless agreed to be a physician leader on the Polyclinic's ICIC experiment largely because of the enthusiasm of his longtime colleague Mark Cordova. "It was probably a full year into the collaborative before I realized that having a system approach was actually going to save me time and result in better care for my patients."

John, Cordova, nurse Colette Rush, and several others from the Polyclinic attended training sessions sponsored by the Washington State Collaborative, at which evidence and testimony was presented regarding improvements in diabetes control achieved via the chronic care model. The sessions broke the model down into its elements and explained their value, including how building computerized disease registries and diffusing responsibility for patients to a clinical team facilitated disease management. John says, however, that he came out of the training unconvinced that any of this was going to make a difference in *his* practice. Indeed, his attendance at the Breakthrough Series and subsequent group discussions might have been for naught if not for an insurance company letter that landed on his desk right around the same time.

The letter, from the insurance company's own quality assurance division, asserted that one of John's patients was overdue for an HbA1c test. "They were notifying me that this patient had not had a hemoglobin A1c in eighteen months," John recalls.

"My reaction was, 'That's ridiculous, of course they did because I know they need it and I would have insisted on it.' But then I checked the chart and the patient hadn't been in to see me in eighteen months," John says. "You know, time flies, and you think you saw them just three months ago but in fact I discovered I really didn't have a way to check on patients who weren't coming in."

Better tracking of patients as well as measurable improvements in their clinical status have made John an advocate of the chronic care model's systematic approach. But he treads lightly in conversations with physician colleagues, remembering his own misgivings about upsetting tried and true practice. He's also mindful of the group practice culture, in which physician autonomy is prized.

"Historically, we were a collection of independent private practices under one roof. In the last ten years, we've been changing—getting more rules and work production and practice guidelines," John says. "I don't resent the clinic suggesting that I do things differently, but some of my colleagues do resent that."

John opts, therefore, to promote the chronic care model via data demonstrating improved medical care quality: "What I tell the reluctant physician is that you are going to do a better job if you use this system," he says.

Health Care Organization: The Polyclinic

As one of the nation's first physician group practices, Seattle's 90-year-old Polyclinic was an ideal setting in which to test the efficacy—and practicality—of the chronic care model. Most Americans get their health care from private physicians in partnerships like the Polyclinic.

Polyclinic leaders had been looking for a way to improve chronic disease management since the late 1990s, when it became clear that managed care and capitation were failing as cost-control mechanisms in Seattle's health care market. "We knew costs were going to go up," says Lloyd David, the clinic's chief executive. And David knew from experience that if costs went up, the purchasers of the Polyclinic's services—health benefits managers for corporations, public employee unions, and the like—would react by trying to "pay less for unit prices."

Not only would that cut into Polyclinic revenues, it also wouldn't accomplish the objective: cost control. When purchasers pay less for an office visit, health care businesses respond by doing less per visit. So patients end up coming in more frequently, pushing costs back up through increased use of services. "So we saw disease management as a means to improve quality and control cost," David says. "It's a win for the patients, a win for the bill payers, and a win for the doctors in improved job satisfaction through improved performance."

The Polyclinic's other goal was to remain competitive as a business. "We were willing to take the risk of spending more up front to save money on the total costs and get paid higher unit costs," David says. Colette Rush, a nurse and longtime case manager, became the clinic's ICIC liaison. She worked from 2001 to 2002 with physicians Gregory John and Mark Cordova to adapt their practices to the chronic care model. "We tracked 220 diabetic patients on seven to eight measures of disease management, and they improved in all measures," Rush says. "We then presented our data to upper management and signed on three more doctors."

By the experiment's second year, the Polyclinic board had seen enough to vote to make the chronic care model clinic policy, though not mandatory, for its primary care physicians. But management turned up the pressure in other ways. The Polyclinic's medical director, Michael Tronolone, says he began issuing quarterly performance reports specific to each of the clinic's thirty-one primary care physicians and based on quality benchmarks for diabetes management, such as annual eye exams and optimum HbA1c results. Physician identities were coded, but it was easy to figure out where each stood in the ranking, according to members of the clinical staff.

"Feedback to the individual is not sufficient to change the system of medical practice," Tronolone says. "It's got to be wide open—performance, compensation, everything. Once you start doing it, it feeds perfectly into what doctors want: to be better than the others or at least not have the others be better than they are." While management used such tactics internally to bring around skeptics, it also began scrutinizing new hires for their ability and willingness to be team players. The objective here was to change the Polyclinic's historically autonomous physician culture. "We don't have a lot of lone wolfs anymore," Tronolone says. "The recruiting message kind of selects them out."

Converting the Polyclinic's diabetics into disease managers was equally time-consuming, according to Nikki Nordstrom, a nurse who is the project's liaison between medical staff and patients. "It was assumed that the physicians would support this, and it was also assumed that patients would be enthusiastic," Nordstrom says. "Truly? It took eighteen months to build acceptance. The theoretical models don't roll out that easily."

Nordstrom says she spent weeks calling diabetic patients to explain the new chronic care system. She emphasized the self-management side of the chronic care model, and invited them to one-on-one educational meetings as well as group seminars on topics such as foot care. "I'd go through all this and the patient would say at the end, "Who are you again? Why isn't my doctor calling me?" Over time, however, patients caught on and began to welcome the attention from others besides their doctors.

"One of the first things we did was tell the patients with diabetes that they had to come in for four visits a year, and that they needed to get their blood work done ahead of time so they could discuss the results with their doctor," Nordstrom says. This helped change doctor-patient dynamics by enabling face-to-face discussion of test results in contrast to a thumbs-up, thumbs-down note in the mail. Physicians also made a point of asking patients to choose their own self-management goals—losing five pounds, say, or adding 100 yards to their daily walk.

Members of the medical staff say clinical results for diabetes have been impressive, leading to a new experiment in secondary prevention for patients with heart disease. And as the Polyclinic lab tallies the evidence of improved outcomes, David, the chief executive officer, is deploying this performance record at the bargaining table, pushing for enhanced fees and year-end bonuses from health insurers if Polyclinic patients stay out of the hospital. He acknowledges the Polyclinic's negotiating advantage as a large and sought-after provider in Seattle's health care market.

"We're able to have a dialogue with the insurers around this issue of reimbursement," David says. "Small practices don't. They just get a take it or leave it letter."

State: Rhode Island

The objective of Rhode Island's ICIC project was to implement the chronic care model statewide over time in all primary care settings. It tested the model in a select group of sites, and succeeded in meeting benchmarks for clinical improvement. But project leaders also discovered how taxing and expensive the process can be, particularly in small medical practices. Rhode Island has few large groups like the Polyclinic. Most physician practices are small partnerships, reflecting the national physician workforce. The state also has a network of community health centers at twenty-six sites, as well as outpatient clinics at its fifteen hospitals. Through collaboration with ICIC, Rhode Island hoped eventually to roll out the chronic care model broadly enough to persuade all primary care practices to move to this standard of diabetes care.

To address the financing side, project leaders invited health insurers to be part of the collaborative. These partners included the state's dominant private insurers, Blue Cross & Blue Shield of Rhode Island and UnitedHealthcare; the quasi-public health plan for low-income families, Neighborhood Health Plan of Rhode Island; and the Medicare oversight commission in Rhode Island, Quality Partners.

"After twenty years in public health, this was the best idea I'd heard," says Dona Goldman, the health department nurse who spearheaded Rhode Island's ICIC project. Goldman, head of the state's Diabetes Prevention and Control Program for more than twenty years, was convinced that standardizing disease management via the chronic care model could significantly improve the health status of Rhode Island's diabetics, whatever their circumstances.

"Initially, there were docs who felt they had nothing in common with health center docs or clinic docs and vice versa," Goldman says. "But if we divide ourselves into the haves and have nots, we can't make this happen, not to mention that we're all paying the price of not doing this better. So I said, 'No, we are not going forward divided.'"

Voting with the majority of ICIC test sites, Rhode Island chose diabetes to test the chronic care model. The reasons were historical, epidemiological, and political. The state health department and community health centers were already working to improve diabetes care under a program sponsored by the Centers for Disease Control and Prevention to reduce health care disparities. One in eleven adults in Rhode Island, or 60,000 people, are diabetic, and health officials estimate that 30,000 more have the disease but don't know it.[6] There has also been an alarming uptick in prediabetic symptoms among teenagers and young adults, suggesting an even heavier burden of illness to come.

The political arguments, however, nailed the case. In order to keep its broad coalition together, Rhode Island needed the hard data on clinical improvement and cost savings that diabetes uniquely delivers. The strategy worked, and diabetes care demonstrably improved at the project's test sites. The evidence was showcased at an outcomes conference in late 2005, including better HbA1c scores and compliance with annual eye and foot exams. Clinicians using the chronic care model to guide diabetes management also testified to learning curves as illuminating as Gregory John's.

But a different set of numbers motivated the behind-the-scenes discussion as Rhode Island's program neared the end of its ICIC funding. To a one, participants questioned the sustainability of clinical improvements without buy-in on health care's financing side. The numbers they wielded illustrated the perverse incentives of the current system. While office visits to monitor and teach diabetics self-management earn fees of $75 to $150, acute events are paid in Rhode Island as follows:

- Hospitalization—$7,285

- Leg or foot amputations—$16,288

- Retinal surgery—$7,420

- Coronary artery disease—$8,020[7]

"There's a lot of potential reward for *not* doing this," says the obstetrician-gynecologist and co-chair of the collaborative, Deirdre Gifford, who thinks the chronic care model underplays the business imperatives of survival. By ditching the patient education and support and seeing diabetics only when they have problems, "you could have a very lucrative practice," Gifford argues.

Heidi Brownlie, a family doctor and chronic care model champion in a five-physician practice, has similar misgivings. "We are finding this very time-consuming," she says. "The practice hasn't bought into this"— by hiring additional staff—"so it is falling on the providers' shoulders. For me, that means I'm taking thirty minutes rather than fifteen with these patients and then I have to cut time with other patients to make up for it."

Having insurers in the collaborative was educational, but yielded no immediate solution to the concerns raised by Gifford, Brownlie, and others. Blue Cross Blue Shield and UnitedHealthcare each made lump-sum donations to augment grant money from ICIC, and more recently began piloting incentive pay formulas with certain physician groups. Beyond that, their efforts have largely been confined to aligning internal monitoring systems with the medical quality standards embedded in the chronic care model. UnitedHealthcare, for example, has built patient education messages into its subscriber website (www.myuhc.com). Both companies also track physician compliance with standards of care, and send reminder letters similar to the one received by the Polyclinic's Gregory John.

Private practitioners aren't the only ones worried about sustaining the chronic care overhaul made possible by ICIC grants. Community health centers are also uneasy, despite an organizational structure in which physicians are salaried and some revenue is guaranteed by government subsidy. The sustainability issue curbed everyone's enthusiasm, even those most excited by the evidence of improved health in their patients. "We only get paid for illness," says Ernest A. Balasco, former executive director of Wood River Health Services. "We pray for good flu seasons, we pray for big allergy seasons, because then our office visits go up and we get reimbursed."

Adds Donna Fantel, Wood River's chronic care coordinator, "In some ways, we are kind of shooting ourselves in the foot by doing this, because we are actually preventing the kinds of visits that are well reimbursed."

—ᴍᴍ— Conclusions

In the early weeks of 2006, the *New York Times* ran a front-page series that neatly framed the mission, the experience, and the wisdom of ICIC.

Published between January 9 and 12, the articles chronicled the escalating toll of Type II diabetes on lives, families, and health care resources. The January 11 installment dealt with the health care system's skewed financial incentives. Headlined, "In the Treatment of Diabetes, Success Often Does Not Pay," the article detailed what ICIC collaborators can rattle off in their sleep: how prevention can be a financially ruinous proposition for health care organizations when insurers fail to adequately cover self-management tools like blood sugar test strips (75 cents apiece), but pay generously for a $12,923 prosthetic lower leg following amputation.[8]

The *Times* series echoed the points made by Lloyd David at the Polyclinic, Ernest Balasco at Wood River Health Center, and Deirdre Gifford of the Rhode Island Chronic Care Collaborative about the difficulty of going forward with chronic care improvements absent a means to pay the upfront costs. And while there has been no dearth of effort nationally to build the so-called business case for improved medical care quality, theoretical projections of future savings aren't cutting it in the current political environment. Public panic over health care affordability has everyone clamoring for savings now.

ICIC grantees had to contend with this political climate. Wagner might be theoretically correct in saying, "Money isn't the problem; misdirected money is the problem," but those implementing the chronic care model had to navigate business environments caught up in the national distress over health care costs. While many physicians, nurses, patient educators, clinic managers, and others enthusiastically endorsed the model's logic, they had a harder time documenting cost savings through better disease management.

The upfront costs, meanwhile, made grantees uneasy. These included salaries for new staff to take on patient education and case management duties, computer upgrades to build disease registries, and expenses associated with being at the leading edge of change. For example, managers said the chronic care model requires training beyond traditional workplace orientation programs to bring new hires into sync with the team approach to patients—investments difficult to justify without clear evidence of payback. The question forever hovered: "How can I sell this to the boss?"

But ICIC's mission wasn't to figure out how to treat people more cheaply. It was to treat them better. In order to do so, the environment of primary care had to be re-engineered to one that was more suited to twenty-first century health threats and remedies. The chronic care model was the means to that end. Reports from the field support ICIC's premise. Clinicians say that utilizing the model makes their approach to chronic patients more proactive, resulting in evidence of improved medical care quality. Patients report greater confidence in self-management and greater support from the medical team.

The questions about financing are valid, but they reflect ICIC's external environment more than they are a substantive commentary on the chronic care model. By metronomic repetition, cost control has so dominated the conversation about health care that worthy experiments in other areas struggle to be heard.

It's the government's job to fix the financing. And the work is under way. Congress and the Centers for Medicare & Medicaid Services—standard-setters in health care financing since Medicare was launched in 1965—are in the middle of a large pay for performance research and demonstration project. There are hundreds of test sites in every imaginable health care setting: nursing homes, hospitals, home health care agencies, dialysis facilities, clinics, and physician practices of every size. Code-named P4P, the government's effort is exploring many of the ideas floated by ICIC grantees to build into health care's financing structure incentives and subsidies to improve medical care. The support from health care leaders is such that just about every A-list health care organization has joined the experiment, including the Joint Commission on Accreditation of Healthcare Organizations, the Agency for Healthcare Research and Quality, the National Committee for Quality Assurance, and the American Medical Association.

By contrast, ICIC seems puny. Nevertheless, its contributions to the collective goal of improving health care are significant. ICIC helped show how the architecture of medical care—office organization, staff deployment, hierarchy, and attitudes toward patients—affects the quality of care. The chronic care model offers a process for changing that architecture so that clinicians and patients can work as partners in managing disease and preventing complications. ICIC grantees demonstrated the model's flexibility by adapting it to a wide range of primary care settings.

This flexibility has applicability beyond current medical practice. If there is a given in today's health care environment, it is the rapid pace of developments in science and technology. In diabetes alone, better drugs and devices for monitoring and responding to changes in blood sugar have dramatically improved the precision with which clinicians and patients are able to manage insulin deficits. Looking ahead, it may soon be possible to intervene at the genetic level, before symptoms even appear. Elias Zerhouni, director of the National Institutes of Health, outlined the promise of ongoing research aimed at such "preemptive" treatment in an interview earlier this year in *Health Affairs.*[9] The chronic care model has the capacity to not only adapt to new science but also to streamline its introduction into clinical practice.

Work remains, however. Among the lingering issues is the slow process of organizational and personal change. The Polyclinic internist Gregory John, now a champion of the chronic care model, says it took him close to a year to let go of professional patterns honed over twenty-five years of medical practice. Nikki Nordstrom, nurse coordinator of the Polyclinic's chronic care team, pegs conversion time at eighteen months for both clinicians and patients. Are there ways to accelerate this?

One answer may come from the next iteration of ICIC—a collaboration with the Association of American Medical Colleges. The goal is to build the concept of proactive team management of chronic illness into medical school curricula and residency training. If the next generation of physicians is educated to expect disease management support for chronic patients, health care organizations will have another incentive to restructure: competition for medical talent.

Another issue is the chronic care model's dependence upon electronic patient records as the structural base for disease registries and population data retrieval. While many medical quality schemes presume a universal patient database, this currently doesn't exist, nor, because of privacy concerns, is there a consensus that it should. Most physician offices in the United States still rely on paper records.

Finally, there is the question of how far ICIC principles of disease management teamwork can extend into the communities where people with diabetes, asthma, and other incurable conditions live and work. Risa Lavizzo-Mourey, president and chief executive officer of the Robert Wood Johnson Foundation, emphasizes the importance of this outreach, saying that she envisions a day when chronic patients are supported in the task of self-management to the degree that those who want to avoid tobacco hazards are aided by public smoking bans.

"Patient-centered care, which is the crux of the chronic care model, essentially comes down to the health system's being oriented to helping patients achieve *their* goals," Lavizzo-Mourey says. "We have to find the baseline elements that cross diagnoses in order to be able to codify systemwide approaches."

Notes

1. Smith, C., Cowan, C., Heffler, S., and Catline, A. "National Health Spending in 2004: Recent Slowdown Led by Prescription Drug Spending." *Health Affairs,* 2006, *25*(1), 186–196.
2. CDC. National Diabetes Fact Sheet, 2005. (http://www.cdc.gov/DIABETES/pubs/pdf/ndfs_2005.pdf)
3. Franklin, W. T., et al. *Report to The Robert Wood Johnson Foundation on Its Programs on Chronic Illness and Aging over the Last Twenty Years,* November, 1992.
4. McCulloch, D. K., Price, M. J., Hindmarsh, M., and Wagner, E. H. "Improvement in Diabetes Care Using an Integrated Population-Based Approach in a Primary Care Setting." *Disease Management,* 2000, *3*(2), 75–82.
5. American Diabetes Association, Diabetes Statistics, 2006. (www.diabetes.org/diabetes-statistics.jsp)
6. Goldman, D., et al. *History of the Rhode Island Chronic Care Collaborative: A Framework for Collaboration.* Presentation to the staff of Blue Cross Blue Shield of Rhode Island, Providence, Rhode Island, April 13, 2005.
7. Rhode Island Department of Health, Center for Health Data & Analysis. *Hospital Community Benefits Data Set,* November 21, 2005.
8. Urbina, I. "In the Treatment of Diabetes, Success Often Does Not Pay." *New York Times,* January 11, 2006.
9. Culliton, B. J. "Extracting Knowledge from Science: A Conversation with Elias Zerhouni. *Health Affairs,* Web Exclusive, 2006, *25*(3), w94–w103. (http://content.healthaffairs.org/cgi/content/abstract/hlthaff.25.w94)

Insurance Coverage

Increasing Health Insurance Coverage at the Local Level: The Communities In Charge Program

Mary Nakashian

Editors' Introduction

Increasing access to health care has been a goal of the Robert Wood Johnson Foundation since its very beginning. In Volume IX of the *Anthology*, Robert Rosenblatt reviewed the thirty-plus-year history of the Robert Wood Johnson Foundation's efforts to expand health insurance coverage to all Americans and concluded that the Foundation's initiatives had oscillated between trying to bring about major change at the national level and working with states and communities to find ways to insure people locally. The Communities In Charge program is an example of the latter approach; it supported fourteen communities' efforts to expand insurance coverage within their limited geographic area.

As Mary Nakashian observes in this chapter, the Communities In Charge grantees ran into many obstacles. These ranged from expected sources of revenue drying up to onerous insurance regulations, and from lack of administrative know-how to September 11th derailing planned activities. As the program unfolded, the communities showed a great deal of ingenuity in meeting the challenges, even if it meant deviating from their original plans. Though the number of people who obtained coverage under the program was disappointing, some of the sites developed strategies that could—and are—being replicated. Communities In Charge and other programs that look to generate local solutions for expanding insurance coverage raise the question of whether efforts to address lack of insurance coverage are best done at the community, state, or federal level, or some combination of the three.

Mary Nakashian, the chapter's author, is a freelance writer and health care consultant. She has served as vice president of the National Center on Addiction and Substance Abuse at Columbia University, executive deputy commissioner of New York City's Human Resources Administration, and in a variety of positions with the Connecticut Department of Income Maintenance.

—ɯ—Nearly 46 million Americans currently lack health insurance coverage, and the number is rising. Between 2000 and 2004, as health insurance premiums escalated and employers cut back on employee coverage, the number of uninsured Americans rose by six million.[1] Lack of insurance has serious consequences for health and well being. Uninsured people often delay getting needed medical care, are in worse health than those with insurance, and encounter financial difficulties paying their medical bills.[2,3]

Four out of five uninsured individuals are employed or live in a family in which the household head is employed, largely in service establishments such as restaurants, hotels, and retail stores. Although two-thirds of uninsured people are white, higher percentages of ethnic and racial minorities lack health insurance. In 2004, 34 percent of Hispanics, 21 percent of Blacks, 19 percent of other races and 13 percent of Whites lacked insurance.[4] Similarly, middle- and upper-class Americans are more likely than low-income people to have health insurance.[5]

More and more people who are employed or who are self-employed find themselves uninsured. People like Sandra Fleming, a self-employed massage therapist from Boulder, Colorado. With income from her massages supplemented by occasional work preparing magazines for publication, Sandra has been able to meet basic expenses. But she cannot afford health insurance. For a while, she was eligible for care at a clinic at a cost of $25 per visit. "I had a mental profile of the people I thought would be at the clinic, but when I walked in, they were different. There were a lot of people who looked like they came to the clinic from work." As her massage practice grew, the clinic had to adjust her fees. "They tell me now I have to pay $73 per visit, and I don't know if I can do that. My payment almost tripled, but my income only went up a little bit."

Over the years, the federal government has taken steps to cover certain groups and to expand coverage. In 1965, Congress passed Medicare, a federal program that covers people over 65 and with disabilities, and Medicaid, a federal and state program that insures poor people. In 1997, it passed the State Children's Health Insurance Program, or SCHIP, a federal-state program that covers children living in low-income families. Proposals for large-scale health care reform surfaced in the Nixon, Ford, and Carter administrations. All of them failed. President Bill Clinton's Health Security plan, proposed in 1993, failed as well.

─ᴡᴡ─ The Development of the Communities In Charge Program

In the mid- to late-1990s, with the failure of the Clinton health plan and national health care reform off the table, the Robert Wood Johnson Foundation turned its attention to states and localities. In contrast to the void at the federal level, states and communities offered promise. State economies were strong, employment was up, and welfare rolls were at historic lows. Anticipating revenue from settlements with tobacco companies, state governments were interested in using those funds to support new health programs in their communities. "Increasingly, the challenge of providing health care to the uninsured was falling disproportionately to local communities," said Judith Whang, the former Robert Wood Johnson Foundation senior program officer who helped develop and monitor the Communities In Charge program.

In attempting to expand health insurance coverage at the local level, the Foundation built upon its experience dating back to the 1980s and a program called Community Programs for Affordable Health Care. This program supported community coalitions in devising ways to manage care and keep medical costs down. Results were disappointing, and in 1990 Foundation officials concluded that the program's central flaw was its misguided assumption that cost containment could be achieved through intervention at the community or local level when the true levers of power existed at the national and state levels of the health care system.[6]

In 1985, the Foundation funded the Health Care for the Uninsured Program to test strategies for making health care coverage more available and affordable to small businesses. Under this initiative, fourteen states either developed new insurance products for businesses or subsidized existing ones. One lesson from this program was that "health insurance, even if heavily subsidized, was unaffordable for small businesses."[7]

In looking for promising community strategies in the mid-1990s, Foundation staff members were encouraged by what they saw emerging in Hillsborough County, Florida, which includes Tampa and surrounding areas. In 1993, the county reorganized the way it financed and delivered health care services to its low-income residents. With a half-cent increase in the county sales tax that had been authorized by the Florida legislature two years earlier, the county government was able to finance Hillsborough HealthCare, a managed care program that emphasized prevention and early detection of health problems. Each year, about 27,000 people received care through one of four networks that operated clinics under contract to the county government. Enrollees received primary and specialty care, hospital services, prescriptions, and vision, dental, and home health care. In 1996, the program won the Ford Foundation Award for Innovations in American Government.

Hillsborough HealthCare interested the Foundation staff because it was an organized system based on primary care and prevention that operated on a large scale and was available to people based on their income rather than on characteristics such as employment or family status. Furthermore, it appeared to be sustainable through ongoing public financing.

As staff members at the Foundation considered how a new program should look, they debated the extent to which it should replicate Hillsborough HealthCare. Although staff members were impressed with the Hillsborough program, they understood that other communities would have different circumstances and priorities and might not be able to replicate what Hillsborough County had done. "We studied the Hillsborough County model to death," recalls Judith Whang. "Early on, we talked about whether it could be replicated. But we decided to focus on strategies that engaged community leaders in designing their own solutions rather than on replicating specifically what happened in Hillsborough County."

In 1997, the Foundation's board authorized $16.8 million for a four-year national program called Communities In Charge. The call for proposals, released the following year, specified that the program was "designed for local communities interested in improving access to care for low-income uninsured individuals by rethinking the organization and financing of local care delivery." It went on to specify that during a one-year planning phase, communities would be expected to:

- Create a process to build consensus regarding funding and service delivery.
- Assess the scope of the problem and resources available to address it.
- Design an actuarially sound financing approach that identifies dedicated and sustainable funds.
- Plan an infrastructure and an information system to administer the development and operation of a managed care system.

To receive three-year implementation grants, communities would be expected to:

- Establish comprehensive delivery networks emphasizing primary care.
- Create detailed implementation plans to operate their projects.
- Design and launch outreach, marketing, and enrollment programs.
- Enroll members and provide services to them.
- Collect baseline and operational data for program management and evaluation.

In 2000, twenty communities received up to $150,000 planning grants. In 2001, fourteen of those communities received up to $700,000 for three years to implement the projects they had planned. Two of the sites (Birmingham, Alabama and Spokane, Washington) later withdrew from the program.

Table 4.1. Communities In Charge Programs and Grantees

Project Name	Location	Program Design
Alameda Health Consortium	Oakland, California	Coverage product for low-income children and their families; new managed care products for low-income adults
District of Columbia Primary Care Association	Washington, D.C.	Expand Medicaid eligibility and enrollment into a D.C.-sponsored coverage program
JaxCare	Jacksonville, Florida (Duval County)	Managed care coverage product with donated hospital services
Community Health Works/ Medcen Community Health Foundation, Inc.	Macon, Georgia	Donated care model providing case management for uninsured with high-risk medical conditions
Project Access/Central Plains Regional Health Care Foundation, Inc.	Wichita/Sedgwick County, Kansas	Donated care model coordinates medical care, prescription drugs, and services
getCare Health Plan (Louisville-Jefferson County Communities In Charge Coalition) (getCare closed in 2005.)	Louisville, Kentucky	Donated care model coordinates access to existing safety net and voluntary specialty care
CarePartners/ MainewHealth	Greater Portland, Kennebec, Lincoln, and Cumberland counties, Maine	Donated care model provides access to health care services, care management and low-cost or free pharmaceuticals
Jackson Medical Mall Foundation/Hinds County Health Alliance	Jackson, Mississippi	ER redirect/disease management program
Brooklyn HealthWorks/ Brooklyn Alliance, Inc.	Brooklyn, New York	Insurance subsidy program
HealthforAll of Western New York, Inc. (HealthforAll closed in 2005.)	Buffalo/ surrounding counties, New York	Insurance subsidy program
Multinomah County Health Department/ Tri-County Health Care Safety Net Enterprise	Portland, Oregon	Regional public corporation for safety net system management and governance
Indigent Care Collaboration	Austin, Texas	Web-based regional information system creation of health financing district

The implementation awards required a dollar-for-dollar match from communities. Virtually all of the communities secured some of their matching funds from the federal Health Resources and Services Administration's Healthy Community Access Program or the W. K. Kellogg Foundation's Community Voices program.

Medimetrix, a health care consulting firm located in Cleveland, directed the program nationally and provided technical assistance to grantees.

—*w*— **Program Implementation**

Even though the Foundation had not required potential grantees to replicate the Hillsborough model, staff members hoped that at least some communities would do so. However, the program diverged from that idea almost from the start. According to Nancy Barrand, one of the original Communities In Charge program officers at the Foundation, "we did not want to say we were replicating the Hillsborough model *per se*—we didn't want to say we were asking communities to pass a sales tax. When the proposals came in, things really morphed. It is common that a program attracts what is out there, not necessarily what you want. For example, we hoped communities would really examine and change the way they financed existing health care and explore ways to reallocate money and reorganize services to make them more effective. But when proposals came in, they suggested more limited initiatives, and we ended up supporting approaches that focused on improving coverage or coordinating care for targeted groups of people such as low-income workers and high users of care. Later, the program morphed even more because of changes in the national economy and fiscal crises in the states. These changes are not necessarily negative, but you should understand why you are getting what you are getting."

The proposals suggested a range of initiatives. Some communities planned to create managed care systems as specified in the call for proposals; some proposed to enroll thousands of new people in existing safety net programs; and some proposed to create new insurance products for working people. In 1999, when community representatives were writing their planning grant proposals, the economy was booming and grantees assumed they would receive approval from the state government to use tobacco-settlement funds for their projects or to tap new funds resulting from a provision in federal law that allowed states to collect higher levels of reimbursement for hospitals that served disproportionate numbers of low-income people. These assumptions generally proved false.

During 2000, after communities received their planning grants, the economy began to deteriorate. By 2001, when projects began their implementation phase, the high employment rates and robust state budgets that characterized the 1990s had evolved into gloomy reports of increasing joblessness and dwindling revenues. After the September 11, 2001 attacks, homeland security became the priority at all levels of government and health care all but disappeared as a concern. These changes forced communities to scale back their original ideas.

As is often the case when community groups attempt to implement new programs, everything took more time than expected. Local grantees did not hire project directors until 2001 when the implementation grants were awarded. Therefore, planning was conducted on a part-time basis by staff members generally employed by one of the health care agencies affected by the project. In some communities, safety net providers were in competition with each other for patients or funds. According to Terry Stoller, the national program director at Medimetrix, "Sadly, the overall funding environment creates a situation where you have local agencies fighting over any community-designated funding crumbs, and you have communities fighting one another over state funding crumbs. Given this mindset, it is not difficult to imagine how challenging it is for these competitors to come together on a project whose goal was to rethink local health care financing and delivery."

Despite tanking economies and nerve-wracking delays, most Communities In Charge projects took hold: As of December 2004, when Foundation support ended, twelve of the original fourteen were still operating. Collectively they leveraged $81 million in public and private funds, enrolled 50,000 people in existing programs such as Medicaid and

SCHIP, and another 30,000 people in programs that were created or expanded through Communities In Charge. One year later, in December 2005, ten of the twelve were still operating.

—ᴟᴟ— Three Communities

Reflecting on the disparate Communities In Charge sites, Anne Weiss, the Foundation senior program officer currently overseeing the program, says, "If you have seen one program, you have seen one program. Each community put its own mark on how it approached and handled everything." While this is certainly true, an examination of Communities In Charge projects at three locations illustrates issues that many sites had to address and the solutions that they adopted. Two of the sites—Brooklyn, New York and Jacksonville, Florida—attempted to make insurance affordable to small business owners and their employees. The third site—Austin, Texas—used new technologies to improve the efficiency of safety net programs.

Brooklyn HealthWorks

Brooklyn is the most populous of New York City's five boroughs with nearly 2.5 million residents. Howard Golden, Brooklyn's powerful borough president for twenty-five years, secured the Communities In Charge planning grant on behalf of his borough. When Golden left office in 2001, one of his parting actions was to hand Brooklyn's nascent Communities In Charge project to the Brooklyn Chamber of Commerce, where it landed on the desk of Mark M. Kessler, the vice president for member services.

Kessler is a former teacher and Peace Corps volunteer. "I'm an incrementalist. I learned to work with what you have, to move the pieces around to make things work. Even so, when we started this, we were not sure we could pull it off, but we wanted to try." Kessler's boss, Kenneth Adams, president of the Chamber of Commerce, adds "We didn't see this as a health care initiative as much as a product that would be useful to our members. We are not health care professionals, but we do know what our members worry about and what they want."

From the start, Brooklyn had two goals for its Communities In Charge project, Brooklyn HealthWorks: first, to create an affordable commercial health insurance product for uninsured businesses with two to fifty employees; and, second, to enroll enough members to ensure its economic sustainability. By the end of 2005, Kessler observed, "Could a local consortium build an affordable, localized commercial health insurance product to meet the needs of its small business community? Obviously, yes. But if such a product was brought to market, would the local small businesses buy it? Not necessarily. We learned that they would not buy products that are 'cheap' but don't work for them. There is a difference between 'cheap' and 'affordable'."

Rosalie Rance runs Viking Hospitality Marketing & Media in Brooklyn. "We develop strategic plans for cultural institutions like museums and tourist destinations like Brooklyn." When she started her business, neither Rosalie nor her sole employee had health insurance. "I was scared to be without coverage and I wanted to offer it to my employee, but it was daunting. I am my own everything—cleaner, secretary, scheduler—and I didn't have time to research and figure out what kind of care I should have, what it costs, where I should get it. I was worried about not having care, but I didn't know what to do about it. I am a member of the Chamber of Commerce and when I found out that the Chamber offered insurance I called Mark. In about ten minutes I understood my options and selected a program. But when I started filling out the paperwork, I learned that there was a lot of other documentation I needed for my business but did not have. This made me go through mounds of paper and work with my accountant to be sure that all my business affairs were in order. Now it is. I have insurance, and I can pay for my employee's health insurance, too. This helps because I want to bring my values to my company, attract good employees and create a stable, supportive working environment."

The Chamber of Commerce took control of Brooklyn HealthWorks early in 2002, began enrolling employers in April 2004 and by December 2004, when the Communities In Charge project ended, had enrolled just twenty-five companies covering 104 employees. When asked about the low level of interest, business owners said the program offered too few providers and those providers who did participate were not located near where workers lived. In August 2005, the Chamber brought Brooklyn HealthWorks into Group Health Incorporated, or GHI, a not-for-profit health insurer that has a network of more than 72,000 providers in New York, New Jersey, and Connecticut. This change solved the provider problem and raised enrollment rates to about 70 people per month. As of February 2006, 157 employers had enrolled, covering 730 workers. "Because it includes a range of providers, the new program offers a better product than our first try. Even though it meant we had to raise premiums, people are buying it because it gives them what they need," says Kessler. While this spike in enrollment is promising, 730 enrollees in a borough with more than 475,000 uninsured people still leaves a lot of people without coverage.

Businesses are eligible to enroll in Brooklyn HealthWorks if they are located in Brooklyn, have between two and fifty employees, thirty percent of whom earn $34,000 or less per year, and have not provided health insurance to employees within the previous twelve months. At least 50 percent of eligible employees must enroll. Brooklyn HealthWorks participants receive an insurance card that entitles them to services through GHI. Employers pay between $177 and $188 per month per employee, about one-third the cost of standard health insurance premiums in New York City. Funds from Communities In Charge and the federal Healthy Community Access Program pay the difference between the employer premium and the full premium cost. Overall, Brooklyn HealthWorks leveraged $2.2 million from other funding sources.

Brooklyn HealthWorks provides coverage for inpatient and outpatient hospital services, physicians' services, maternity care, adult and child preventive health care, x-ray and lab services, emergency services, and other named services. For companies that choose the more expensive premium, employees pay a co-payment from $10 to $20 a visit. The prescription drug program has a $100 deductible per year and a $10 co-payment per generic drug.

Jonas Kyle and Miles Bellamy, owners of Spoonbill and Sugartown, Booksellers, purchased Brooklyn HealthWorks for themselves, their spouses, their children, and two of their three employees. "For a while, my kids got care through Child Health Plus"—New York State's health insurance plan for children—"but then when my wife went back to work, we didn't qualify for that anymore, and no one had insurance. This has been especially important for my kids. My daughter got hurt and we had a doctor who would see her, and now we have a regular doctor" says Kyle. "She would not have had care if we didn't have Brooklyn HealthWorks."

People who participate in Brooklyn HealthWorks love it, so why did it take so long to launch a program that serves only 730 people? It certainly wasn't for lack of hard work. Among the things that happened were the following:

- While the events of September 11th rippled across the country, they virtually halted life as usual in New York City for some time.

- The Chamber of Commerce had to satisfy a complex maze of New York State Insurance Department regulations and secure approval to become part of a larger New York State health insurance initiative, Healthy New York. In the end, these systems fell into place and actually improved Brooklyn HealthWorks, but the administrative work took more than one year.

- After state regulatory issues were resolved and despite GHI's commitment to Brooklyn HealthWorks, negotiations over premium rates, benefit packages, and claims processing systems took an additional fifteen months.

- When the Chamber of Commerce initially approached businesses about purchasing health care for their employees, most were interested. When it came time to enroll workers, however, both employers and workers were less enthusiastic, partly because the roster of providers participating in Brooklyn HealthWorks was so small before the program became part of GHI's provider network. Also, according to Kessler, "While many employers tell us they are interested in providing coverage to their employees, when it comes time

to make a decision, many simply cannot afford to do so and
may not want to admit it."

- Moreover, employees in the lowest-wage jobs (less than about
$11 an hour) asked that employers give them the value of the
health premium in the form of wage increases rather than
health coverage. This caused some tensions between business
owners who thought they were being generous in purchasing
health care for employees and the employees who felt that
their need for additional income outweighed their need for
health insurance.

- Fifth, because New York City has a strong public health
system, people have health care options that low-income
people in other parts of the country generally do not have.

The Brooklyn experience appears to reinforce the lessons learned from
the Foundation's earlier programs aimed at small businesses—they don't
work. So, why try again? National program director Terry Stoller notes,
"We were worried about projects that focused on small businesses because
we knew about earlier, unsuccessful efforts to interest business owners to
purchase insurance. But we also knew that Brooklyn had a lot of the elements that seemed to be lacking in other places. It had a strong political
champion, an attractive and comprehensive product costing one-third the
price of competing products, solid project management, a smart marketing
campaign, and a small geographic area that included thousands of potentially eligible businesses and employees. The fact that, even with all of these
powerful attributes, Brooklyn had so few employers in its program should
dissuade other communities from using this approach."

Kessler and the Brooklyn HealthWorks staff are not so sure. "One
thing we learned through this is that you can't innovate on a schedule.
What breakthrough ever happened in the timetable people set at the
outset? We had a lot of design and start-up problems, but since August
2005, we have been steadily enrolling more than 70 people per month,
and there is no reason, except for funding, that won't continue. If we
expanded Brooklyn HealthWorks citywide, based on our current enroll-

ment of more than 70 people a month in Brooklyn, we estimate we could enroll more than 10,000 additional people."

"Kessler may have a point. In July 2006, the New York State Legislature appropriated funding of $2 million annually to expand HealthWorks in New York City and to add a new HealthWorks initiative elsewhere in the state."

JaxCare

With a population of 774,000 spread over 758 square miles, Jacksonville looks very different from Brooklyn, but it also has its share of uninsured people. Nearly 14 percent, or more than 100,000 Jacksonville residents, lack health insurance.

As was the case with most Communities In Charge locations, Jacksonville entered the planning phase with a noble vision and great hopes. It used its Communities In Charge planning grant to prepare to add 10,000 people to an existing low-income health care program. The planning group intended to pay for this expansion with $10 million in new city funds and newly designated state funds available for hospitals that provide a disproportionate share of services to people without insurance coverage. But the group was not able to secure city and state buy-in for such a significant investment and was forced to abandon this strategy just as the Communities In Charge implementation phase was due to begin.

Enter Rhonda Davis Poirier, a health care consultant with a doctorate in public health and a reputation for getting things done. According to John Delaney, Jacksonville's mayor at the time, "She is a 'never-say-die' person. I think most of us who were involved were really skeptical, but she wouldn't give up."

Under the sponsorship of the Jessie Ball duPont Fund, headquartered in Jacksonville, and Communities In Charge, Poirier co-convened a series of eight health policy forums. These forums were created to educate key city leaders about health care issues concerning the uninsured in Jacksonville and to secure consensus about JaxCare's design. The mayor and the presidents of all of Jacksonville's hospitals personally attended these three-hour meetings and the monthly working sessions in between.

By the end, all were convinced that the policy forums were the key to making JaxCare work. A. Hugh Greene, president and chief executive officer of Baptist Health and the chairman of JaxCare's board of directors, says, "What the forums did was to 'create the table.' The table is the engagement of key stakeholders. I was amazed that everyone kept coming. We had our disagreements. Once, one of the very important leaders got up and walked out. I literally ran after him, caught him at the elevator, and convinced him to come back. I think if he had gotten on that elevator and left, we would have lost the others too." Sherry Magill, president of the Jessie Ball duPont Fund adds, "This was a serious project for our community and for my organization. Neither of us wanted to fail, and we did not want to fail in front of the Robert Wood Johnson Foundation."

Poirier notes, "Through these meetings, we built a common understanding of the facts and challenges of providing care to uninsured people in Jacksonville. The forums provided an opportunity and a framework for community leaders to communicate candidly with each other about these issues. And JaxCare's current board of directors includes many of these same people who are still actively engaged and regularly attend board meetings."

By the end of 2002, forum members had reached agreement on a pilot program that would serve 1,600 low-wage workers. The City of Jacksonville committed $2.5 million, which local hospitals matched with in-kind services or funds. JaxCare also received a federal Healthy Community Access Program grant and funds from local corporations and foundations. In all, JaxCare leveraged $6.5 million in outside funds.

JaxCare was ready to go, pending final confirmation from the state that the program was exempt from regular state insurance requirements. Despite earlier assurances to the contrary, this turned out to be a problem. State officials ruled that JaxCare had to secure an insurance license and comply with all state requirements governing health insurance—requirements that the project could not meet. Everything stopped. Finally, after Governor Jeb Bush intervened, Duval County, in which Jacksonville is located, was added to Health Flex, a state program for low-income people that operated outside of regular insurance regulations. Waiting for the State's initial decision and then applying for approval under Health Flex rules delayed JaxCare's implementation by nine months.

In 2003, JaxCare became a non-profit 501(c)(3) organization headed by Poirier. It provides health care to low-income workers between 19 and 64 years old living in Duval County who have been uninsured for at least six months, have been working for the sponsoring business for at least ninety days, have household incomes less than 200 percent of the federal poverty level, and are not eligible for government-sponsored health insurance programs.

Between 50,000 and 60,000 workers are eligible for JaxCare coverage, which includes primary and specialty physician care, generic pharmaceuticals, inpatient and outpatient hospital care, diagnostic services, and disease-management services. Businesses pay $50 per month for each enrolled employee, and the employees pay a $15 monthly premium. This is about 20 percent of the actual cost of the JaxCare premium. Enrollees are assigned a primary care physician from among the more than 900 physicians who participate in the program, and they receive hospital services from the hospital where their primary care physician has privileges.

Henry Osborne left a career as an aide to former Florida Senator Lawton Chiles and the Secretary of the Department of Business and Professional Regulation to return home to Jacksonville where he purchased North Florida Scrap Metals, a company that buys discarded machinery, extracts metals from them, and resells the metals. "I didn't know the business when I started, but I learned. I'm so much happier using my hands and I'm fitter than I've ever been!" Early in 2004, Henry secured health care for his three employees through JaxCare. "When I came here, no one had insurance. I asked an insurance agent about purchasing care for my employees, but I couldn't afford it. I heard about JaxCare and called right away, and all of my guys qualify for it. To me it was a no-brainer."

JaxCare began enrolling businesses in March 2004 and by December 2005, 122 employers and 389 employees had signed up, far short of the 1,600 goal. At the beginning, JaxCare focused only on small businesses—those employing three or four workers. In order to increase enrollment, the program launched a marketing blitz aimed at large employers who already covered some, but not all, of their employees. The theory behind this strategy, which has not been widely tested, is that the chief executive officers of these companies have already made a decision to provide insurance as a matter of policy and will be amenable to extending coverage to all their employees. Floyd Willis, a family practitioner at Jacksonville's Mayo Clinic, president of the Duval County Medical Society and a member of JaxCare's board of directors, notes, "Sometimes when we call company leaders, they have no idea that some employees don't have coverage. We are the ones telling them their employees are showing up in emergency rooms because they can't get care elsewhere because of the lack of coverage. We learned that often, when we talk directly to the CEO's, they motivate and give direction to their staff. It didn't work when we started with mid-level management in the companies."

Like Brooklyn HealthWorks, JaxCare has struggled to gain enrollees, and for many of the same reasons. "Start-up was a lengthy process and when we thought we were all set, the state's decision regarding our insurance status meant we had to abandon implementation and focus exclusively on getting state approval. We lost a lot of momentum when that happened," says Poirier, echoing the experience described by Mark Kessler in Brooklyn. "Even now, with the program up and running, we have to navigate a complicated maze of state regulations and adhere to state policies that limit our ability to enroll people. For example, we have enrolled 122 businesses, but two to three times that number have chosen not to enroll because we can't offer JaxCare to all of their employees, only the ones who meet all our eligibility guidelines. Because small business owners know each of their employees, they are just not prepared to offer a benefit like this to some but not other employees who need it just as much. Changing the income guidelines requires state legislation. The Florida legislature has shown little interest in amending these laws for us, despite the fact that there is no state money involved and we have the support of our local health care and health insurance industries."

Poirier, however, is still a believer. "We have all the necessary systems in place and are fully operational," she says. "We have more than enough physician and hospital capacity, and we have the unmet need. We could easily expand our administrative infrastructure to serve a much larger number of people."

Austin, Texas

The population of Travis County, Texas, which includes Austin and surrounding towns, rose from more than 576,000 people in 1990 to nearly 870,000 in 2004—a 51 percent increase. About 200,000 people, or nearly 23 percent of county residents, do not have health insurance.

In 1997, before Communities In Charge began, executives of twelve Travis County safety net health care providers, including several hospitals, clinics and the medical society, formed the Indigent Care Collaboration, or ICC, to improve the financing and delivery of health care to all residents of the central Texas region. They established the ICC with the explicit expectation that it would design and oversee strategies to improve their ability to serve patients or reduce their costs. Diana Resnik, a senior vice president at Seton Healthcare Network, known as the "whirling dervish" of health care in Austin, spearheaded the creation of the ICC. Staffed by Resnik and other volunteers, the ICC was incorporated as a not-for-profit 501(c)(3) organization in 1998.

Safety net providers, worried about the growing number of uninsured people in the county, looked to the ICC for help. "I had been meeting with colleagues for years and we talked about the situation, but we couldn't do anything about it except cry and make each other feel better," said Resnik. "So my boss asked if the ICC could do something. I agreed to try, but I said to him, 'You have to be there. The big guys won't come for me.' So with my chief executive at the table, the other CEOs came as well. In addition, the reason the ICC members stayed engaged was our commitment to action. We were not willing to meet and just talk. We knew we wanted to work on a uniform health care screening tool, and we wanted to find a way to share information with one another. When we heard about the Robert Wood Johnson Foundation program, we knew what we wanted to do."

According to Paul Gionfriddo, project director of the Travis County Communities In Charge project from April 2001 until May 2005, "We didn't do a new product like some of the others because we couldn't afford to. Estimates showed it could cost as much as $350 million to cover everyone. Our thinking was that if we couldn't afford the product, we would have to work with what we already had." Patricia Young Brown, president and CEO of the Travis County Hospital District and chair of the ICC board of directors, adds, "We started with projects that were important to people who were paying the bills and providing the care. We also knew from the start that we needed to raise public money and get an ongoing funding stream. So we started exploring the possibility of creating a hospital taxing district in which a portion of property taxes would be dedicated to health care."

Although the opportunity to participate in Communities In Charge was attractive, leaders of Austin's health care community were initially reluctant to apply. Mildred Vuris, director of governmental and community relations at the Austin Travis County Mental Health Mental Retardation Center and one of the original members of the ICC, recalls, "Some people said, 'This is too hard, too much work. Do we want anyone from the outside controlling what we do?' I said, 'Yes we do!' And so we agreed to apply." Concerned that an application featuring only one county would not be well-received by the Robert Wood Johnson Foundation and because many people who work in Austin live in adjacent Williamson and Hays Counties, the ICC opened its membership to those counties as well.

When the ICC received the implementation grant, it hired a full-time project director, Paul Gionfriddo—a former state legislator, mayor, and executive director of a non-profit organization. With the Foundation's and the federal Healthy Community Access Program's funds in hand and an experienced leader on board, the ICC got to work. It used the Communities In Charge funds to create a range of technology-based tools that would give its members comprehensive online information about their patients and help low-income people obtain coverage through existing programs such as Medicaid and SCHIP. As people moved from uninsured to covered status, providers would be reimbursed for services, thereby increasing their revenue and reducing the burden of providing uncompensated care. In quick succession, the ICC:

- Launched "Medicaider," an online tool for staff members in health care settings in the three counties to screen patients for eligibility for federal, state, and local health coverage.

Medicaider takes about three minutes to complete, and people who appear eligible for coverage receive assistance in completing their applications and obtaining benefits. As of November 2005, of the more than 215,000 people screened using Medicaider, 42,000 had been found eligible for an existing public program. Providers who use Medicaider agree to pay for it because it saves them money when their patients have coverage.

- Created I-Care, a Web-based database to store patient-specific health information contributed by each ICC member. I-Care captures data such as zip code, age, gender, and ethnic background of patients served by clinical programs. It also gives participating providers online information about diagnosis and procedure codes for patients' prior medical visits. I-Care complies with the strict federal and state privacy rules required by the Health Insurance Portability and Accountability Act (HIPAA). As of November 2005, I-Care contained information on more than 1.8 million patient encounters and 440,000 individual patients.

- Initiated Project Access, patterned after a project in Asheville, North Carolina, in which physicians volunteer their time to provide free care to needy patients. As of September 2005, the more than 850 physicians participating in Project Access had served 1,165 patients.

- Expanded annual Dental Sealant Days, during which more than 450 children receive free dental screenings and dental sealants.

- Created a pharmacy assistance program that enabled uninsured and indigent patients to gain access to free and subsidized drug programs offered by pharmaceutical companies. From its inception in June 2004 through November 2005, nearly 2,400 people received a total of

> 15,400 free prescription drugs that, if purchased, would have
> cost $4.3 million.

In total, Travis County leveraged $5.3 million in federal, state, local, and private funds to support these efforts.

When Hurricane Katrina stormed through Louisiana and Mississippi, many residents fled or were evacuated to Texas. About 7,000 were temporarily housed at Austin's convention center. The ICC quickly discovered that many evacuees had serious medical needs and had left their homes without essential prescriptions or medical equipment. While some evacuees had private or public health insurance, virtually no one could document that they had coverage. According to Kit Abney, director of "insure a kid," a community collaborative that screens people for government-funded health care coverage and assists them in enrolling, "As a result of the relationships and protocols established by our Communities In Charge project, Ann Kitchen, the executive director of the ICC, pulled together the safety net providers on a conference call, and right away we came up with a system for helping evacuees living in Austin find a doctor and get care. All the providers said they would waive eligibility; my office became the hot line and referred people to the provider closest to them and the one best positioned to meet their health care needs. The medical society developed a specialty care line to get people to specialists, and we worked with the people to make sure they could get to their appointments."

In May 2004, Travis County voters authorized a "countywide hospital district to furnish medical aid and hospital care to indigent and needy persons residing in the district." The new hospital district is financed by a levy added to property taxes paid by people who live in Travis County and provides some funds to the ICC.

Ann Kitchen, a social worker, attorney, former state legislator, and health policy expert, who took over the ICC in May 2005, says, "We have a lot of challenges ahead, including sustaining funding and improving the user friendliness of the I-Care technology. We are also beginning new projects that will take our Collaboration to the next step. For example, we are creating a disease-based management program for patients with chronic conditions such as diabetes or mental illness. These patients tend to require care from multiple providers, and often no one sees the whole picture. With our Web-based registry, providers will be able to get that picture. We have also started a project to determine the real gaps in physican services in our region. We know we do not have enough primary and specialty care physicians, but we also know we can do better with what we have by being more efficient."

Travis County's approach has generated interest elsewhere in Texas and across the country. In 2004, after consulting with ICC staff, health care providers in San Antonio created the "Access to Care for the Uninsured" collaborative to address the needs of San Antonio's uninsured residents. With assistance from Kitchen and others at the ICC, this group applied for and secured a $950,000 federal Healthy Community Access Program grant to create a tool like Medicaider and a program for sharing patient information, much like I-Care. In Florida, Paul Gionfriddo, now the head of the Palm Beach County Community Health Alliance, is replicating many of the strategies developed in Travis County: a Medicaider eligibility screening tool, a system of shared information based on I-Care, and a Project Access network where volunteer physicians provide care to needy patients. "The truly remarkable thing about what happened in Austin is that it does appear to be a transportable model," says Gionfriddo. "And the people who sustain it are the people who will benefit from it."

—᙭— Communities In Charge in Retrospect

With nearly $17 million of Foundation funds and $81 million of leveraged funds, the twelve Communities In Charge sites enrolled only 30,000 people in new health care coverage programs. If the measure of success is coverage of new people, the program clearly did not succeed.

The picture improves somewhat, however, if the measure of success is expanded to consider whether people who enrolled in existing or new coverage programs as a result of Communities In Charge received preventive and primary care. The Communities In Charge evaluation, led by the University of Michigan economist Catherine McLaughlin, found that in the three communities it surveyed—Austin, Texas, Alameda County, California, and southeastern Maine—there was a noticeable increase in physician visits, and an even larger increase in the number receiving physical exams, Pap smears, and breast exams.[8] In Austin, for example, the percentage of women having had a breast exam rose from 22 percent in the year before enrolling in the program to 51 percent within a year after enrolling; 30 percent reported having had a Pap smear within a year prior to enrolling and 62 percent said they had a Pap smear within a year after enrolling. Only 28 percent of enrollees said they had a physical exam in the year prior to enrolling, while 59 percent had an exam within a year after enrolling. These findings raise the possibility that because people were receiving preventive care, health problems might have been detected earlier and treated more inexpensively than would have otherwise been the case.

If the measure of success is further expanded to include whether grantees produced useful products and strategies, certainly some did. National program director Stoller said, "If you look at Travis County, they created a relatively inexpensive, successful, and replicable set of strategies. Things like that are real accomplishments." Similarly, the policy forums in Jacksonville offer an innovative method of changing the way safety net providers make decisions. While created specifically to plan for Jacksonville's Communities In Charge project, the forums continue to bring together a group of powerful health care and political leaders who talk with knowledge and broad understanding about health policy.

Robert Wood Johnson Foundation senior program officer Anne Weiss says, "Certainly, Communities In Charge didn't yield the vast new numbers of covered people that we hoped for. But just because those things weren't what we were looking for at the outset, we should not miss the many good things that did happen. For example, that Travis County voters authorized basically a new taxing mechanism to pay for indigent care is not a small thing."

By 2002, the Foundation's priorities had shifted from supporting community-based efforts to expand coverage to encouraging expansion of health insurance at the national level. "We concluded that we did not lack for solutions," says Weiss. "What is lacking is the national will to make the kinds of changes that would be necessary. The Foundation made a decision to invest future funds and efforts into creating that will."

Evaluator Catherine McLaughlin offered a similar observation on the lack of potential of community programs to expand coverage. "What I saw twenty years ago when we were evaluating a program in Rochester, New York, what I saw ten years ago in Hillsborough County, and what I see now is that a lot of this is luck," she said. "In Rochester and Hillsborough, the stars were all in alignment—the right people were in place, the need was urgent, and funds became available. These community innovations are anomalies and it is not reasonable to expect that what they did can be done anywhere else or at any other point in time. To the extent that financing and regulation are not local, it is naïve for community leaders to think that they can do this."

Mark Kessler, of Brooklyn HealthWorks, has a different perspective. "I understand that we need a national will. Certainly Brooklyn HealthWorks is not going to solve the entire problem," he said. "At the same time, I don't think it's wise to focus so much on creating the will. That could take a long time and while it might benefit future generations, our business owners, their employees and their children all lack insurance now. And we can't ignore them while we wait for the will. We have to do both."

Notes

1. Kaiser Commission on Medicaid and the Uninsured. *Covering the Uninsured: Growing Need, Strained Resources.* Menlo Park, Calif.: Kaiser Family Foundation, November, 2005. (www.kff.org/uninsured /7429.cfm)
2. Institute of Medicine, "It Is Now Time to Extend Coverage to All." *Project on the Consequences of Uninsurance: An Overview.* Washington, D.C.: Institute of Medicine, 2004.
3. Starr S. S. and Fernandopulle, R. *Uninsured in America.* Berkeley and Los Angeles, Calif.: University of California Press, 2005.
4. *Cover the Uninsured Week,* Facts and Figures, April, 2006. (www. covertheuninsured.org/factsfigures)
5. Ibid.

6. *See* Schroeder, S. A., Cohen A. and Cantor, J. "Perspectives: The Funders." *Health Affairs,* 1990, *9,* 29–33.

7. Rosenblatt, R. "The Robert Wood Johnson Foundation's Efforts to Cover the Uninsured." *To Improve Health and Health Care, Vol. IX: The Robert Wood Johnson Foundation Anthology.* San Francisco: Jossey-Bass, 2006.

8. Taylor, E. F., McLaughlin, C., Warren, A., and Song, P. "Who Enrolls in Community-Based Programs for the Uninsured, and Why Do They Stay?" *Health Affairs,* Web Exclusive, 2006, *2(3),* w183–w191. (http://content.healthaffairs.org/cgi/gca?sendit=Get+All+Checked+Abstract%28s%29&gca=25%2F3%2Fw183)

The Partnership for Long-Term Care: A Public-Private Partnership to Finance Long-Term Care

Joseph Alper

Editors' Introduction

For many Americans over 65, gaining access to high-quality long-term care has proven to be a formidable challenge. The Robert Wood Johnson Foundation's efforts to improve access to and quality of long-term care includes programs to improve nursing homes;[1] to expand home care, adult day care, and assisted living;[2] to give elderly people more choice in the type of care they receive;[3] to encourage volunteerism,[4] and to better integrate the delivery of medical care and long-term care[5] among other initiatives.[6]

Then there is the problem of paying for long-term care. The cost of nursing home care routinely impoverishes older Americans, who are then forced to rely on Medicaid (or to spend down in order to qualify for Medicaid). Long-term care insurance, a way of protecting people against going broke in old age, is expensive and has appealed primarily to a narrow band of upper middle-class or wealthy individuals. To increase the appeal of long-term care insurance, the Robert Wood Johnson Foundation, in 1987, initiated an experimental program called the Program to Promote Long-Term Care Insurance for the Elderly. This program fostered a new and controversial type of long-term care insurance product that allowed nursing home patients with state-approved private long-term care insurance policies to be eligible for Medicaid with substantially higher levels of assets than are normally allowed. This would permit them to receive nursing care and still have enough to live on and to bequeath to their children.

Joseph Alper, a freelance journalist and frequent contributor to The Robert Wood Johnson Foundation *Anthology,* describes the logic of the program and the hurdles that had to be overcome to field the demonstrations, including federal legislation limiting the program to the four states. The result of nearly twenty years' effort is mixed. The product has proven viable, but the number of policies sold to date—especially those sold to middle-class and lower middle-class individuals—is far smaller than was expected. The story ends on an upbeat note, however, with the passage of legislation in 2006 that will allow all fifty states to market the private-public policies.

1. Bronner, E. "The Teaching Nursing Home Program." *To Improve Health and Health Care, Vol. VII: The Robert Wood Johnson Foundation Anthology.* San Francisco: Jossey-Bass, 2004.
2. Henry, R. S., Cox, N. J., Reifler, B. V., and Asbury, C. "Adult Day Centers." *To Improve Health and Health Care 2000: The Robert Wood Johnson Foundation Anthology.* San Francisco: Jossey-Bass, 1999.
3. Benjamin, A. E. and Snyder, R. E. "Consumer Choice in Long-Term Care." *To Improve Health and Health Care, Vol. V: The Robert Wood Johnson Foundation Anthology.* San Francisco: Jossey-Bass, 2002.
4. Dentzer, S. "Service Credit Banking." *To Improve Health and Health Care, Vol. V: The Robert Wood Johnson Foundation Anthology.* San Francisco: Jossey-Bass, 2002; and, Jellinek, P., Appel T. G., and Keenan, T. "Faith in Action." *To Improve Health and Health Care 1998–1999: The Robert Wood Johnson Foundation Anthology.* San Francisco: Jossey-Bass, 1998.
5. Alper, J. and Gibson, R. "Integrating Acute and Long-Term Care for the Elderly." *To Improve Health and Health Care 2001: The Robert Wood Johnson Foundation Anthology.* San Francisco: Jossey-Bass, 2001; and Begley, S. "The Covering Kids Communications Campaign." *To Improve Health and Health Care, Vol. VI: The Robert Wood Johnson Foundation Anthology.* San Francisco: Jossey-Bass, 2003.
6. Mockenhaupt, R. E., Lowe, J. I., and Magan, G. G. "Improving Health in an Aging Society." *To Improve Health and Health Care, Vol. IX: The Robert Wood Johnson Foundation Anthology.* San Francisco: Jossey-Bass, 2006

—ɯ— One of the great economic changes that has occurred over the past twenty-five years is that the United States has become a nation of investors. Over two-thirds of Americans now own their homes, and for many of us our home is our biggest investment. Just over half of all households own stock, thanks to the availability of mutual funds and tax-favored retirement vehicles such as 401(K) plans. The median net worth of the average American household now stands at just over $100,000, and is just under $200,000 for Americans age sixty-five and older.[1]

But looming on the horizon is something that could not only strip those assets from a great many American households but also draw significant financial resources from both the federal treasury and state government coffers. That "something" is the need for services to help individuals suffering from a chronic physical ailment or deteriorating mental capacity—a broken hip, signs of dementia, a car accident, any medical condition that requires long-term care.

"Every American is at risk of needing long-term care, and for most middle-class Americans that means that all of the assets that they've worked a lifetime to accumulate are at risk," says David Guttchen, director of the Connecticut Partnership for Long-Term Care. "At the same time, as the baby boomers age, the growing need for long-term care that will occur has the potential to overwhelm the Medicaid system and place a huge burden on state budgets." Joyce Ruddock, a vice president at MetLife in Connecticut, adds, "This is a problem that we as a nation are going to have to face, and the sooner we do it, the better individuals will be and the better our government's finances will be."

Long-term care expenditures represent one of the largest medical and financial risks facing elderly Americans today. While we all want to believe that we will remain healthy and active until dying peacefully in our sleep at night, the harsh reality is that nearly half of all Americans turning sixty-five years of age will spend time in a nursing facility at some point in the remaining days of their lives. Given that the average cost of a year of long-term care was $72,240 in 2004 and that the average length of long-term care is two and a half years, it is easy to see that an economic train wreck awaits many unprepared Americans. A few Americans, mostly members of the upper-middle class, have purchased long-term care insurance—relatively expensive coverage that under specified conditions provides skilled nursing or custodial care in a nursing facility or at home following an injury or an illness. Most Americans, however, either cannot afford or choose not to buy long-term care insurance and are at risk of suffering catastrophic expenses if they need long-term care.

But individuals are not alone, because state and federal Medicaid budgets are on that same train, heading for the same financial disaster. Today, long-term care accounts for a third of Medicaid funding. From 1990 to 2003, Medicaid spending on long-term care increased from $30 billion to $87 billion, costs shared by state and federal governments.[2] With Medicaid already accounting for more than 20 percent of state spending, state budgets could be as overwhelmed by long-term care costs as the typical American's pocketbook would be.

Charles and Gloria Dougherty are manifestly not in the ranks of the unprepared. Charles, sixty-five, and Gloria, his wife, fifty-nine, have each purchased a long-term care insurance policy that enables them to protect $182,000 in assets and pay for five years of nursing home and home care benefits. If either Charles or Gloria requires more than five years of care, Medicaid would then assume the ongoing costs, even though the couple would still have their nest egg. "This is the best way to protect ourselves," Dougherty says.

Before the Dougherty's bought long-term care insurance, their plan, like that of many middle-class Americans, had been to transfer their assets to a relative if either husband or wife needed long-term care, and then apply for Medicaid assistance. An individual with more than $2,000 in nonhousing assets is normally ineligible for Medicaid services, and anecdotal evidence suggests that a growing number of Americans are planning to essentially bankrupt themselves and then apply for Medicaid if they should need long-term care. Congress has, however, made it increasingly difficult for middle-class families to spend-down, qualify for Medicaid, and have the government pay for their long-term care. Medicare, to the surprise of most people, covers little in the way of long-term care expenses.

The Doughertys, though, are among the 225,000-plus Americans who have taken advantage of a unique program to insure themselves against having to hide their assets if they do require long-term care. This program, the Program to Promote Long-Term Care Insurance for the Elderly—also known as the Partnership for Long-Term Care—was initiated in 1987 with funding from the Robert Wood Johnson Foundation and has been offering asset-protecting long-term care insurance policies in California, Connecticut, Indiana, and New York. Since the early 1990s, private insurance companies have been selling special Partnership policies that have protected approximately $30 million dollars in assets while saving the states an unquantified amount of money—but an amount that state officials nonetheless say is significant.

Since 1992, fewer than 150 policyholders out of more than 250,000 have exhausted their benefits and applied for Medicaid. "It doesn't take much of a leap to see that these policies are protecting the states from a much bigger number of Medicaid claims," says Sam Morgante, vice president of government relations at Genworth Financial in Washington, D.C. Genworth, the successor to GE Financial's insurance business and AMEX Life Assurance Company, is the country's leading seller of long-term care insurance.

Connecticut's Guttchen, along with his colleagues in California, Indiana, and New York, agrees wholeheartedly. "Can I tell you exactly how much money Connecticut has saved? No. But has the state saved money? Absolutely," Guttchen says. Michael Staresnick, who heads Indiana's Partnership program, estimates his state's savings at $2.2 million over twelve years. "Is that a huge savings? No, but it is a savings nonetheless, and given the challenges we've faced in getting people interested in long-term care period, let alone in buying Partnership policies, we're encouraged that this program will save us substantial dollars over the coming decades."

—w— A Novel Partnership is Born

State governments have been eager to head off the impending avalanche of long-term care claims against their Medicaid programs. Indeed, the states woke up to the magnitude of the problem in the mid-1980s, and it was their explorations into how long-term care insurance could help both their treasuries and their citizens that helped lead the Robert Wood Johnson Foundation to launch its Partnership for Long-Term Care initiative in 1987. The idea of the program was to work from concepts that several national and state commissions, as well as social policy experts, had developed through meetings and studies:

- Delaying the moment at which patients qualify for Medicaid—which occurs when patients exhaust their assets or spend them down to the maximum level allowed for Medicaid eligibility—could avoid financial disaster among long-term care patients and their families.

- Preventing such spending down could also save public funds.

- An overwhelming majority of Americans believe it is wrong to transfer assets and want to take personal responsibility for funding their long-term care.

- Elderly consumers would benefit if risk pooling—special programs created by state legislatures to provide a safety net for medically uninsurable populations—could be implemented.

Though the Foundation's formal role in this program ended a decade ago, the experiences of California, Connecticut, Indiana, and New York have finally gotten the attention of Congress. In February of 2006, President George W. Bush signed into law a bill that will allow the remaining forty-six States and the District of Columbia to create their own Partnership programs. This will enable Americans to share the responsibility of paying for long-term care with state and federal governments while making it harder for them to shield their assets before turning to Medicaid to fund a part of their long-term care.

"Congress has finally recognized the successes of the Partnership programs and has taken the necessary steps to open these plans to all Americans, not just those lucky enough to live in the four states with existing programs," says Stephen Somers, a former associate vice president and program officer at the Robert Wood Johnson Foundation, who founded and heads the Center for Health Care Strategies, in Hamilton, New Jersey. "The result will be a win-win-win-win situation because individuals, insurers, and both state and federal treasuries will all come out ahead thanks to the expansion of this program."

This is exactly the outcome that the Foundation had hoped for when it started the Partnership program, says Mark Meiners, director of the Center for Health Policy Research and Ethics at George Mason University in Fairfax, Virginia. Meiners headed the national program office that oversaw the program when it was based at the University of Maryland, and he still holds monthly conference calls with state officials administering the current Partnership programs.

According to Meiners, the goal of the Partnership program was to fund the efforts of interested states to develop strategies that would encourage middle-class Americans to buy private long-term care insurance, and to provide an incentive to do so by including some form of asset protection. These policies would then enable individuals to shoulder a significant part of the burden of providing for long-term care while shielding the states from a majority of the cost of paying for long-term care for a growing number of people.

"Private long-term care insurance was certainly available when we started the Partnership program, but the plans were expensive, often confusing, didn't always protect assets, and were usually deficient in terms of consumer protections," Meiners says. "These policies were somewhat successful with the wealthiest Americans, but wealthy people don't usually think about Medicaid, and so these early long-term care polices weren't addressing the issue of how to finance long-term care for the majority of our citizens in a fiscally responsible manner.

"Our intention with the Partnership program was to work with interested states and insurance companies in true partnerships to explore different avenues for making private long-term care insurance more appealing and affordable to the middle-class public. The idea was that if we could design high-quality insurance products and get the insurance industry to sell those policies at a reasonable cost, significant numbers of middle-class Americans would take advantage of this opportunity. The result, at least in theory, would be that individuals would take more responsibility for their own care while enabling the states' Medicaid programs to act as the safety nets they were designed to be and not a *de facto* long-term care program."

In response to the Foundation's initiative, eight states—California, Connecticut, Indiana, Massachusetts, New Jersey, New York, Oregon, and Wisconsin—received planning grants to define and develop a public-private insurance partnership to pay for long-term care. These states explored a variety of ideas on how to encourage the use of long-term care insurance to help their citizens avoid impoverishment, but the basic approach of the four states that eventually created long-term care insurance programs—California, Connecticut, Indiana, and New York—was the same, and that approach involved giving consumers a new choice: buy a state-qualified insurance policy and get special asset protection in exchange for shouldering some of the responsibility for their long-term care.

Normally, when a conventional long-term care insurance policy runs out, policyholders risk having to spend virtually all their savings before qualifying for Medicaid. But by buying a Partnership policy, a person qualifies for Medicaid benefits under special rules that each of the four states established with the approval of the federal Medicaid agency and that the remaining forty-six states will now be able to duplicate. As a result, when a Partnership policy is exhausted, the policyholder is permitted to retain predefined levels of assets that depend on the specific policy purchased, which in turn depend on the state in which the individual lives. The person thus becomes eligible for coverage under Medicaid without having to be impoverished.

"By including asset protection in the Partnership policies, we've created a product that for a relatively small price becomes an important financial tool that an individual can use to protect all that he or she has saved over a lifetime," says Adrianna Takada, director of New York State's long-term care insurance program. "Middle-class Americans today purchase all kinds of insurance to protect themselves and their savings."

She adds, somewhat wistfully, "Now if only we could get more people to think about long-term care insurance in the same way."

—ᴍ— A Long and Winding Road

In 1987, when the Robert Wood Johnson Foundation initiated the planning phase of its Partnership initiative, long-term care insurance was a rather new and expensive product, and most consumers took the attitude that this was something that they either couldn't afford or didn't understand and therefore weren't interested in buying. "In the early days, long-term care insurance was something we sold largely to upper-middle-class and wealthy individuals, with little emphasis on the middle class," says John Greene, senior director of federal affairs for the National Association of Health Underwriters, or NAHU, a professional organization that represents insurance agents. "Partnership plans have changed the situation dramatically."

The idea that the Foundation would play a role in redesigning long-term care policies so that they would appeal to the middle class—and therefore get the middle class to shoulder part of the responsibility for providing for their long-term care if they should need it—began in 1986, when James Knickman, who was then a professor of public policy at New York University's Wagner Graduate School of Public Service, and Nelda McCall, who was then at SRI International, an independent think tank in Palo Alto, California, convened a meeting that brought together leading thinkers in the health care financing field and social policy experts to discuss ideas on how to head off the looming long-term care crisis. Through a series of meetings held in the fall of 1986 and the spring of 1987, Knickman, McCall, and others refined their ideas and attempted to overcome some fundamental disagreements between those who believed that government should shoulder all of the burden for long-term care through a new entitlement program or an add-on to Medicare and those who favored a hybrid model requiring American citizens to take on some of the responsibility for their long-term care needs. In 1987, Knickman and McCall met with Jeffrey Merrill, who was then a Foundation vice president, and Somers, who was a Foundation senior program officer at the time. "Jeff and Steve ended up being the real driving forces that got the Partnership program funded and running," Knickman says.

The process of designing the Partnership program fell to Meiners and his deputy, Hunter McKay, who has since moved to the Department of Health and Human Services. They began their efforts by getting in touch with officials in eight states that had demonstrated a commitment to reforming long-term care financing. As part of the planning phase, the eight states collected data from nursing homes, the elderly population, state Medicaid files, and insurers to help them design and price their products and to assess the products' impact on costs. The data confirmed the idea that a hybrid approach would best balance the needs of the nation and middle-class Americans. "We realized that there was a compromise position, one in which the insurance industry and state governments would share the risk of paying for long-term care protection, and by doing so insurance companies would be able to offer policies that were far more affordable to the average American, and to increase the market for their products," Meiners says.

The three guiding principles that came from reaching this conclusion were that:

- Insurance companies would offer policies with comprehensive coverage but for a limited time and with a limited maximum payout that would be equal to the dollar value of assets that a consumer wanted to protect.

- The states would then provide Medicaid coverage for all policyholders once they had exhausted their benefits.

- The policies would contain consumer protection provisions assuring worthwhile coverage.

For example, an insurance company might sell an individual a policy that paid out a maximum of $200,000 over a three-year period; such a policy would protect the assets held by the average American age sixty-five or older and cover the average two-and-a-half-year length of long-term care. The insurance company would assume the risk inherent in providing that amount of coverage, with the state assuming the risk that the policyholder would require lengthy long-term care. By sharing this risk, the insurance company could sell its policy for a reduced premium, making such policies more attractive to Americans of average means. The states, in return, would assume the responsibility and associated risk of paying for care beyond three years while being shielded from the risk that large numbers of their citizens would divest assets and apply for Medicaid benefits immediately. Part and parcel of this partnership was the notion that consumers would take personal responsibility for a significant part of their long-term care, with the reward of being able to legally protect the assets that they had worked hard to acquire.

Unfortunately, the whole concept of asset protection was not allowed under Medicaid rules, and it appeared that Congress would have to pass legislation that would allow states to approve such policies. "Given that there were certain powerful legislators who were totally against anything but a federally funded program [to pay for long-term care], it appeared that the Partnership program was dead in the water," Somers says. "That was when the Connecticut team came up with what in retrospect was a brilliant solution, and then the Partnership program was off and running."

—⁓— It Pays to Read the Regulations

"It was 1990, and the Robert Wood Johnson Foundation gave us an ultimatum," Connecticut's David Guttchen recalls. "Either we figured out an alternative to Congress's changing the Medicaid rules or the program would end."

The House of Representatives had just voted down a bill that would have allowed the states with planning grants to proceed with Partnership program demonstrations, and the Foundation was set to change course and spend its money on more fruitful endeavors. Kevin Mahoney, who was then Guttchen's boss in Connecticut, pored over the regulations and found a provision that would allow for asset protection with a simple amendment to the state's Medicaid plan. Amendments to state plans are common, and require only signoff from the lawyers at what was then called the Health Care Financing Administration and is now the Centers for Medicare & Medicaid Services. The Foundation hired a Washington, D.C. law firm to write an opinion on Connecticut's plan amendment, and with that legal blessing Mahoney asked the state's newly elected governor, Lowell Weicker, to sign a letter requesting HCFA approval for the necessary Medicaid plan amendment.

"To his credit, the governor-elect signed the letter, and in January, 2001, we received formal approval to go ahead with the Partnership demonstration," Guttchen says. Within months, New York, California, and Indiana received official approval to amend their state Medicaid plans, and the Partnership programs were off and running, with California, Connecticut, and Indiana trying one approach to asset protection and New York taking a slightly different tack.

The Partnerships in California, Connecticut, and Indiana were based on what is known as the dollar-for-dollar model. Under the dollar-for-dollar model, for every dollar of long-term-care coverage that the consumer buys from a private insurer participating in the Partnership, a dollar of assets is protected from the spend-down requirements for Medicaid eligibility. The individual buys a policy that stipulates the amount of coverage. That figure is also the amount that the insurer will pay out in benefits under long-term care coverage when the policyholder is admitted to a nursing home or is receiving long-term care at home or through community-based services.

At the point at which that amount paid out by the policy is equal to the amount of the policyholder's assets, Medicaid can assume coverage, following application for Medicaid eligibility. However, the policyholder must contribute any income to pay for the coverage. With non-Partnership policies, Medicaid coverage would begin only when the insured had spent down nonhousing assets to approximately $2,000. However, with Partnership policies, special Medicaid eligibility regulations allow the policyholder to keep assets up to the level of insurance-paid benefits.

For instance, assume that a purchaser wants to protect $100,000 in nonhousing assets. The purchaser would buy from a Partnership insurer a policy to cover that amount. When the policyholder becomes eligible for benefits either by being admitted to a nursing home or by receiving long-term care at home or through community-based services, the insurer will cover those expenses up to $100,000—or up to the total of the policyholder's remaining nonhousing assets, if those assets happen to fall below $100,000. After that sum is paid out by the insurer, the policyholder must spend down remaining assets to $100,000, at which point Medicaid coverage can begin, pending application to Medicaid and a determination of eligibility. The policyholder is allowed to keep the $100,000 in nonhousing assets—in addition to the approximately $2,000 everyone is permitted to keep—though any income received, such as Social Security, pension, or income from nonhousing assets, must be contributed to the policyholder's care.

The New York Partnership was based on a different model, known as the total-assets protection model. In this type of plan, certified policies must cover three years in a nursing home or six years of home health care, or a combination of the two (with two days of home care equal to one day of nursing home care). Once the benefits are exhausted, the Medicaid eligibility process will not consider assets at all. Protection would be granted for all assets, though an individual's income must be devoted to the cost of care.

Partnership policies in each of the four states also included significant consumer protection features, including five percent compound inflation protection and required agent training. "One of the issues with long-term care insurance is that you're buying coverage that you may not use for twenty to thirty years, and without inflation protection, that $100,000 in benefits you purchased when you were sixty may get you very little when you're eighty and actually need nursing home care," says Raul Moreno, a research specialist with the California Partnership for Long-Term Care.

Each of the implementation states conducted extensive promotional and educational campaigns designed both to inform the public about the Partnerships' policies and to increase sales. Assistance for some of these campaigns was funded by Robert Wood Johnson Foundation communications contracts with public relations firms. The states also collected and analyzed sales and marketing data, and have used the information to evaluate the Partnership programs and make changes as needed and allowed.

For example, Indiana has now added a total assets protection option to its policies, while New York revamped its program to add a dollar-for-dollar provision. New York has also added a tax credit for Partnership policy premiums. "Our initial product was bad," Brenda Bufford, chief of California's Partnership for Long-Term Care, acknowledges. "But we redesigned the policies in terms of adding some consumer protection provisions and getting rid of benefit caps and other provisions that experience showed us weren't working, and now Partnership policies are solid products that [insurance] agents want to sell to middle-class Californians."

—ᴗᴗ— Grinding to a Halt

It wasn't long before officials at the four states with demonstration projects came to the conclusion that the Partnership program offered real opportunities to get consumers to take responsibility for their eventual long-term care needs. "Once individuals heard about the Partnership policies, either from one of the informational meetings we were holding or from an insurance agent, they were far more likely to actually buy a policy," Guttchen says. And agents, according to both NAHU's Greene and Genworth's Morgante, loved selling the policies. "The Partnership policies quickly became a favorite with agents, because they came with a sort of state seal of approval and because they opened up an entire new market for long-term care policies—the middle class," said Greene.

Soon other states were making plans to establish their own Partnership programs. "While each of the four demonstration projects had its own limitations, the general feeling was that we were definitely on the right track," Meiners recalls. "Certainly, we were getting lots of calls from the states looking for information and help in the days after the first four states were up and running."

Not everyone was happy with the end run that the Partnership programs had made around the Congress, however. "At the time, there were certain powerful members of the House who really felt that Partnership policies would primarily benefit the rich," said Katherine Hayes, a senior staff member in Senator Evan Bayh's office. Bayh was supportive of Indiana's Partnership program when he was the state's governor, as was Robert Orr, who was governor when the state received its first grant in 1988.

As a result, Congress included language in the Omnibus Budget Reconciliation Act of 1993 (OBRA 1993) that specifically required states to recover assets from the estates of all persons who have received services under Medicaid. While OBRA 1993 did grandfather the four states that had already created their Partnership programs, for all intents and purposes the language spelled the end for any program not yet running. "While states obtaining a state plan amendment after that date are allowed to proceed with Partnership programs, they are also required to recover assets from the estates of all persons receiving services under Medicaid," Meiners says. "The result of this language is that the asset protection component of the Partnership is in effect only while the insured is alive. After the insured person dies, states must recover what Medicaid spent from the estate, including protected assets.

"At the very least, this becomes a very complicated and convoluted message for consumers. It also removes one of the major incentives people have to plan for their long-term care needs. The effect has been to significantly stifle the growing interest in replicating the Partnership in other states. Promising efforts in Colorado, Illinois, Iowa, Maryland, Michigan, and Washington, to name a few, were sidetracked by the impression that Congress did not support this program."

The proverbial silver lining in this congressional storm cloud was that California, Connecticut, Indiana, and New York were able to run their Partnership programs largely out of the public eye. "Once OBRA was passed, it gave the four [grandfathered] programs a chance to establish themselves, to tinker with the details of how each state tailored its program to meet the goals of increasing uptake of long-term care insurance among the middle class, and to actually gain some experience with what was certainly an experimental program," said Melanie Bella, who helped get Indiana's Partnership program started and has since joined the Center for Health Care Strategies.

The states learned, for example, that inflation protection was a critical feature, and all Partnership policies include five percent compound inflation protection. Indeed, this has proved so popular that many non-Partnership policies now include this provision. Partnership states also put a significant amount of effort into developing objective measures of disability in order to determine what would trigger policy benefits to begin. The four Partnership states also created mechanisms and actuarial standards with which to review initial premiums and any subsequent request for premium increases, which by and large participating insurers have not requested. "Because of the objective procedures we put in place with our Partnership program, it has become far more difficult for companies to justify premium increases, and that has created stability that we think has helped sell long-term care insurance overall," Guttchen says.

—〰— Assessing the Effort

From more than a dozen interviews with state government officials, congressional staff members, insurance industry executives, and social policy financing experts, there seems to be little agreement as to whether the Partnership experiment has proven to be a success, even one with limited scope. On the one hand, there are those such as Nelda McCall, who evaluated the Partnership program for the Foundation. "Was the program perfect? No, but in retrospect I would say that it was a success as far as it went, given that it never got a chance to go beyond the four initial states," McCall says. Meiners adds, "We're at a point now where I think we can say that the four states have tweaked their Partnership programs with experience and have worked out the kinks, and we can now safely say that the program saves costs."

Those who question the program's success raise several points. First, they say it is too early to claim that the program is saving the government money. "We don't have enough experience yet to judge," says Judy Feder, dean of the Georgetown Public Policy Institute. "And I think that when you look at the cost of these policies, they haven't dropped enough to convince middle-class Americans that long-term care insurance makes sense for them." Stephen Moses, president of the Center for Long-Term Care Reform in Seattle and an outspoken critic of involving the Medicaid program in long-term care, concludes, "After a decade of trial, the consensus of thoughtful analysts and critics is that the Partnership has failed to achieve its main objectives."[3] He says, "All this [program] does is perpetuate the idea that eventually Medicaid will bail individuals out of the financial crisis that results from needing long-term care. Medicaid is going broke—it's not going to be here when the limited benefits available under the Partnership policies run out. The Partnership program would be far more successful if the link with Medicaid was severed."

But the most glaring failure, critics say, is that contrary to the designs of the program, the majority of those who bought Partnership policies were in the upper rather than lower income groups. Data gathered in the mid-1990s found that in the states that offered the plans, Americans in the middle-income and lower-income groups bought more standard long-term care policies than Partnership policies.[4] "I believe that this type of data, along with the fact that not many people actually bought Partnership policies, says that the program failed the market test," says Joshua Weiner, an expert on long-term care and health economics at RTI International in Washington, D.C.

Even supporters of the program agree with Weiner on that last point. "If there is one thing negative to say about the Partnership program, it's that the number of policies sold isn't that large, given the sizable populations of the four states that have Partnership programs," Bella says. Joyce Ruddock, of MetLife, concurs: "You can list a lot of reasons why we haven't sold as many Partnership policies as we would have liked to, but the bottom line is that we've come up short so far, though I expect that going forward we, and by we I mean both MetLife and the insurance industry, will be renewing our efforts to sell Partnership policies."

What is the reason that so few Partnership policies have been sold to date? At the top of everyone's list is a lack of sufficient marketing oomph. "We've lacked the resources to market this program as widely as we would have liked," says Michael Staresnick, the head of Indiana's program. "And because the Partnership program was limited to four states, I don't think the insurance companies had the incentive to put significant resources into marketing these policies, either." Connecticut's Guttchen adds, "With long-term care insurance, you're already in a hole, because the fifty-year-olds that we want to reach aren't interested in hearing about long-term care and the problems it can cause them financially, and if you don't have the educational effort to really get that message out constantly, in many venues, and from many sources, you're never going to get that many people to buy long-term care insurance of any kind."

Another reason may be cost. Marc Cohen, a vice president of Life-Plans, Inc. and president of the Center for Health and Long-Term Care Research, wrote, "The average premium of Partnership policies selling in 1996 was 25 percent higher than the premiums of other long-term care insurance policies and 13 percent higher than other policies selling in Partnership states. Thus, that fewer moderate income individuals can afford the policies is not surprising."[5] Moreover, it may be, as Weiner has written, that people do not really care about protecting their assets and want to avoid Medicaid, rather than have easier access to it.[6]

The states also underestimated the importance of getting the insurance agents excited about Partnership policies. New York's Takada says. "We needed to take charge of agent training and really explain to the agents the benefits of the Partnership policies compared with traditional long-term care policies."

John Greene of NAHU agrees that insurance agents haven't played as big a role as they could have in getting the word out about Partnership policies, but he expects that to change dramatically going forward. "The Partnership states have done a tremendous job creating a very good product over the past ten years of running their programs, and what we're hearing from our members is that they are now chomping at the bit to sell these policies to their clients," he says. Morgante of Genworth, adds, "We have big plans now for making a major marketing push for Partnership policies."

Ironically, the impetus for this newfound excitement about Partnership policies comes from Congress, whose members have now been swayed by data compiled by the insurance industry, required as a condition of their ability to sell Partnership policies. For example, the sale of long-term care policies in Partnership states has grown an average of 7 percent over the past five years compared with no growth in non-Partnership states. But perhaps more important, of those individuals who bought long-term care insurance, those buying Partnership policies have a lower net worth than those buying non-Partnership policies.

"We've found that most of the Partnership policies we've sold are to middle net worth individuals," Morgante says.

And according to Katherine Hayes, these data, combined with the fact that each of the four Partnership states believes it is saving Medicaid dollars, led former foes of the program to remain neutral during the past year's debate over legislation that will allow the remaining forty-six states to offer Partnership policies. "There's also the realization that long-term care costs are rising rapidly and that here is a program aimed at the middle-class that protects both consumers and public funds that experience has shown can work," she says. "Is it a panacea? No, but the members of Congress now see it as program with no real downside." John Greene, who spent a great deal of time lobbying for congressional action on the Partnership program, adds, "This is now seen as an apple pie kind of program that hits all the right buttons—it encourages personal responsibility, it depends on a strong public-private partnership, and it doesn't cost the government a dime."

Notes

1. Bassett, W. F., "Medicaid's Nursing Home Coverage and Asset Transfers." *Federal Reserve System Report 2004-15.* Washington D.C.: U.S. Federal Reserve, 2004.
2. Kaiser Commission on Medicaid and the Uninsured. *Medicaid and Long-Term Care,* May 2004. Menlo Park, Calif.: Kaiser Family Foundation, 2004. (www.kff.org/medicaid/7089a.cfm)
3. Moses, S. A., "The Long Term Care Partnership: Why It Failed and How to Fix It." In *Who Will Pay for Long Term Care? Insights from the Partnership Programs.* Chicago: Health Administration Press, 2001.
4. Ibid.
5. Ibid.
6. Weiner, J. M., "The Limits of the Partnership for Long Term Care." In *Who Will Pay for Long Term Care? Insights from the Partnership Programs.* Chicago: Health Administration Press, 2001.

Services for
Vulnerable Populations

Supportive Housing

Lee Green

Editors' Introduction

In this chapter, freelance writer and journalist Lee Green traces the Foundation's investments in housing from early efforts to provide health care services to homeless people to its current support of the Corporation for Supportive Housing, which provides both housing and ancillary medical and social services to formerly homeless people. Foundations such as Robert Wood Johnson, Ford, and Pew Charitable Trusts have adopted supportive housing as a way of assisting homeless people, as have government entities such as the federal Department of Housing and Urban Development and the Department of the Treasury's Community Development Financial Institutions Fund program.

The chapter illustrates the breadth of the interventions that the Robert Wood Johnson Foundation has undertaken in its efforts to improve the health of the American people. While it is fair to ask why a foundation devoted to improving health and health care should support housing programs, Green clarifies the relevance of housing to health and traces the linkage of the Foundation's supportive housing efforts to its earlier mental health initiatives. This linkage is particularly important since many homeless or formerly homeless people suffer from psychological or addiction problems.

Supportive housing offers a prime example of the Foundation's work to improve the medical and social services received by vulnerable populations. Grants to support direct services comprise the heart of what the Foundation calls its vulnerable populations portfolio and its commitment to support hands-on efforts to improve the care offered to society's most needy people.

—ɯ—Lafayette Square, a seven-acre park just across Pennsylvania Avenue from the White House, has long attracted homeless people. A homeless veteran who used to camp out there had a sign that read, "I see you not looking." The homeless people who come to the park lie on benches or sprawl on the grass as tourists across the barricaded street pause along a black wrought-iron fence and gape at the presidential residence. The iconic symbol of American power and prosperity juxtaposed against a park where the nation's most downtrodden languish offers ironic contrasts that cannot be ignored: power and powerlessness, wealth and poverty, haves and have-nots. On a winter night in 1984, Jesse Carpenter, a sixty-one-year-old Army veteran who had been homeless for twenty-two years, froze to death in Lafayette Square. Forty years earlier, on a World War II battlefield in Brittany, France, he had carried three wounded men to safety under heavy fire and later received a Bronze Star for his courage.

—ɯ— Ending Chronic Homelessness

On a cool morning in November, 2004, Lafayette Square lay wet and empty. The homeless had gone elsewhere earlier to seek refuge from a light rain. A few blocks east, in a thirteenth-floor auditorium at the National Press Club, six representatives of America's institutional campaign against homelessness were issuing a landmark proclamation. Nine partners, including the Robert Wood Johnson Foundation, the Conrad N. Hilton Foundation, the Rockefeller Foundation, Fannie Mae, the Fannie Mae Foundation, the Melville Charitable Trust, and Deutsche Bank, would step up "to galvanize leadership and dollars" not just to make a dent in the problem but "to bring an end to long-term homelessness over the next decade."

The goal was breathtaking, but the plan was simple: these organizations, calling themselves the Partnership to End Long Term Homelessness, would eliminate chronic homelessness in ten years by contributing more than $37 million in grants and loans toward establishing 150,000 units of supportive housing—permanent housing with on-site support services—across the nation. Bearing responsibility for using that money wisely and implementing the strategy on the ground were the two remaining members of the Partnership: the National Alliance to End Homelessness, an advocacy organization that seeks to mobilize society's nonprofit, public, and private sectors in a concerted effort to eliminate homelessness, and the Corporation for Supportive Housing. Together, these players, through their own efforts and those of other organizations inspired by their example, would lead the way toward creating a society in which Jesse Carpenter never would have frozen to death anywhere, much less within a few hundred yards of the White House.

Underscoring the seriousness with which the coalition took this ambitious goal was the presence in the room of the president, chief executive officer, or board chairman of each of the participating organizations. They sat on the dais, a long table draped in starched white linen with royal blue bunting, and one by one each rose to address the media. Risa Lavizzo-Mourey, the Robert Wood Johnson Foundation's president and chief executive officer, followed Gordon Conway, who was then the Rockefeller Foundation president, to the podium.

"Supportive housing really must be a part of the safety net that we have in this country to end chronic homelessness," Lavizzo-Mourey declared. "It's not enough for us to put our financial capital in. I think all of us at this table are committed to putting in our reputational capital, our intellectual capital—in other words, in leveraging all of our resources to end chronic homelessness."

Not that anyone in the Partnership even remotely suspected that the organizations at the table could do it alone. Carla Javits, president and chief executive officer of the Corporation for Supportive Housing, or CSH, later laid it on the line: "Really, the intent is to galvanize more investment from businesses and foundations and others—to say, 'We're putting up something as a challenge to all of you to do even more, but this is not enough. It's going to take more than this.'"

Ending chronic homelessness is a dizzying challenge. Ending it in a decade is even more dizzying, given how entrenched homelessness has become in our culture. The Partnership wasn't the first to publicly promote such a goal. Over the past few years, it seems, everyone from Congress to the Millennial Housing Commission to the President's New Freedom Commission on Mental Health has declared that America will end its chronic homelessness within a decade. Depending on when they made their proclamation, some of them are further into that decade than others.

But can social change in any society occur that quickly? Representative Barney Frank of Massachusetts, speaking extemporaneously to Partnership members at a private luncheon following the Washington press conference, expressed doubts about the adequacy of federal funding in a governmental era marked by strong resistance to tax increases. Frank's comments contrasted with the unbridled determination of his audience. They also contrasted with the sunny outlook of Philip F. Mangano, executive director of the United States Interagency Council on Homelessness, who in a May 2002 interview published in the street newspaper *Spare Change News* conveyed big-picture optimism, citing historic sociopolitical upheavals in the United States, South Africa, and the Soviet Union that, once begun, ran their course quickly. "If slavery can be undone in seven years, if apartheid can be undone in seven years, and if totalitarianism in the Soviet Union can be undone in seven years, I have a firm belief that here in America, with all of our resources, with all of our good will . . . we can undo the social evil of homelessness in the same way," Mangano said.[1]

The beginning of a solution involves appreciating the magnitude of the problem, and counting the homeless has always been problematic. Where do you find people who have no home? How do you find those who have no wish to be found? How do you count a population in constant flux? How, for that matter, do you define homelessness?

Estimates vary, but a reasonable likelihood is that between 2.3 and 3.5 million men, women and children in the United States will experience a period of homelessness in a given year. As many as 250,000 individuals and 30,000 families find themselves homeless not for brief intervals but for long stretches.[2] They have spent years caroming among temporary shelters or between shelters and the street. These people, invariably hampered by mental illness, substance abuse, HIV/AIDS, or some combination of those or other afflictions, constitute the chronically homeless. While they account for a relatively small proportion of the homeless population—probably no more than 10 or 15 percent—their demands on hospital emergency rooms, drug clinics, shelters, ambulances, paramedics, psychiatric facilities, police, jails, prisons, and other public social services exert an enormous drain on the system at great expense to local, state, and federal treasuries. Experts posit that this group of troubled individuals consumes a hugely disproportionate percentage of the resources devoted to homelessness.

"I think it's an embarrassment that we have this problem," Lavizzo-Mourey said not long after the Washington press conference. "But I think that the fact that people in both the private and public sectors have identified it as something that we can't allow to continue speaks to the hopefulness of where we're going with this."

—ɷ— Supportive Housing as a Possible Solution

One of the keys, Lavizzo-Mourey believes, is supportive housing, which represents not only a humane solution but probably a cost-effective one as well. Studies in many different parts of the country have all come to the same conclusion: making supportive housing available reduces formerly homeless people's use of shelters and hospitals and time spent in jail. It may save money as well. According to a 2002 University of Pennsylvania study, which was partially funded by the Corporation for Supportive Housing and is considered the gold standard on the subject, placing a mentally ill person in New York City in supportive housing adds just $995 per year to the $40,449 it costs that individual to remain homeless and repeatedly rely upon the institutional safety net of hospitals, emergency rooms, mental health facilities, jails, prisons, and the like.[3] But even the $995 differential is misleading, the study's authors point out, because their analysis did not include savings that supportive housing confers by reducing the burdens on the police and courts. Nor did it assess the economic impact of homelessness on local businesses and tourism. Or on city, state and federal policymakers and staff that devote time and resources to ongoing homelessness issues and to the uneasy relationship between the homeless and the rest of society.

Greater efficiencies may be realized as the supportive housing model is improved and refined over time, but the reduced strain on many of our social institutions is immediate. The University of Pennsylvania study found that in the course of a year a homeless person with severe mental illness typically spends seven weeks in hospitals and nearly three weeks in jail or prison. That's in addition to two months in psychiatric hospitals and 4.5 months in shelters. When the formerly homeless live in supportive housing, hospital beds are freed up, overcrowded jails are relieved, and hospital emergency rooms become less burdened.

—⁓— The Robert Wood Johnson Foundation and Homelessness

Though the Robert Wood Johnson Foundation's mission is to improve the health and health care of all Americans, experience has taught the organization that to be in the health business it also needs to be in the housing business.

"If you think about the way that our health care system is organized, one has to have a residence in order to really gain access to the system in any kind of meaningful way—in order to set up appointments or to get follow-up care, in order to have a coordination of services," Lavizzo-Mourey says. "It all really presumes that you've got a place where people can contact you and coordinate those services. Just being able to do anything beyond an acute visit becomes very difficult if you don't have a home, a place of residence."

The Robert Wood Johnson Foundation's awareness of the inextricable link between housing and health care dates back at least to the early 1980s. The Foundation, in conjunction with the Pew Charitable Trusts, launched Health Care for the Homeless, its first large national program involving homelessness, in 1985. The objective was not to house the homeless but rather to increase the availability of health care services to them. The seven-year program put health care in shelters in thirteen cities and was a model that helped pave the way, in 1987, for Congress's passage of the Stewart B. McKinney Act, which created a federal funding stream for health services for the homeless.

"The lesson from it was that you can't expect homeless people to go to health care sites the way other people do," says Stephen Somers, a former Foundation associate vice president who oversaw the program during its final years, and is now president of the Center for Health Care Strategies. "You've got to bring health care to them. So you set up special clinics and mobile vans and you go under bridges in order to get care to them. And it isn't just medicine and medical care, it's mental health, substance abuse services, food and shelter, you name it."

Health Care for the Homeless was one of the first Foundation-funded programs to shift the focus from traditional models of health care to "other social services critical to a person's health and health status," Somers says. "It just opened the door a little bit."

"We were overwhelmed by the needs," recalls Nancy Barrand, a senior program officer who oversees the Foundation's relationship with CSH. "And one of the biggest needs was mental health care"—a recognition that led, in 1985, to the Foundation's Program on Chronic Mental Illness. This nine-city initiative represented the Foundation's first foray into housing.[4] It was not a housing program *per se*—in fact, housing was but a small piece of it—but it zeroed in on people with serious mental illness, Barrand says, "who just happened to also be homeless." The housing component represented "the recognition that it's very difficult to treat these people and provide them any continuity if they don't have a place to live."

What was at work here was not just care directed to individuals but systems change. Housing was crucial, but housing was expensive. Somers knew his way around Washington, D.C., having worked for Senator John Heinz of Pennsylvania and, before that, for the U.S. Department of Health, Education and Welfare. He looked up old acquaintances at the Department of Housing and Urban Development and suggested that they channel Section 8 housing vouchers, which subsidize housing for low-income people, into the program. HUD did just that, "and so the housing feature of the Program on Chronic Mental Illness became a very important feature of a program that otherwise would have been almost pure mental health care," Somers says.

In the meantime, the Foundation wanted to expand its efforts to improve the health care of homeless people. The Health Care for the

Homeless Program focused on single adults, especially men, because at the time they were the face of homelessness. That program's successor, the Homeless Families Program, began in 1989 and concentrated mainly on homeless mothers with children, more and more of whom were showing up at shelters.[5] With the availability of Section 8 vouchers from HUD, the Homeless Families Program placed much more emphasis on housing as part of the intervention. It had become increasingly clear that the shortest distance between the homeless and health is housing. That may seem obvious now, but in the 1980s Americans were still figuring it out.

—ⱳ— The Corporation for Supportive Housing

The largest Robert Wood Johnson Foundation program addressing health care for the homeless is one that has at its core the sustained and evolving efforts of the Corporation for Supportive Housing or CSH. In fifteen years, CSH has grown from mere concept to a highly focused organization with offices in California, Connecticut, Illinois, Indiana, Michigan, Minnesota, New Jersey, New York, Ohio, Rhode Island, and the District of Columbia. Since December of 2000, when Carla Javits became CSH's president and chief executive officer, Oakland, California, where Javits is based, has served as the *de facto* national headquarters. Recognizing that it can expand to other regions without expanding its brick-and-mortar presence, CSH also works on targeted initiatives in Colorado, Kentucky, Maine, Oregon, and Washington.

But merely establishing that the organization does its work in fifteen states and Washington, D.C., understates the influence CSH has managed to achieve in its relatively short institutional lifespan. Functioning as a national resource center, CSH responds to individuals and organizations from throughout the country, giving them the best available advice on how to navigate the financial and bureaucratic labyrinth confronting anyone trying to develop supportive housing for the chronically homeless. Quite likely, no entity knows more about the subject or has a better big-picture grasp of the inherent complexities than CSH. Every year, the organization hosts a national conference that draws about 150 participants from around the country.

None of this activity would particularly matter if nothing were getting done on the ground, but since its advent, CSH has steered more than $1 billion from public-sector and private-sector donors into projects that have created 15,000 units of supportive housing. That means that 15,000 people with all sorts of mental and physical ills and addictions and social inabilities, people who in many cases spent years on the streets, often revolving through a kaleidoscope of acute relief, shelters, and temporary housing, now have a permanent home. They also have a measure of security, privacy, and dignity that once seemed beyond their grasp. As 2005 drew to a close, CSH had 10,000 more units "in the pipeline," Javits says, and had played a key role in facilitating a landmark November, 2005, agreement between New York City and New York state that promised $1 billion in public funds to create 9,000 more units in New York City alone. "There has never been an initiative that big to develop supportive housing," Javits says.

The term "supportive housing" did not exist in 1990, when a thirty-one-year-old woman named Julie Sandorf asked the Foundation to help fund the creation of a new organization. A year earlier, she had been running a program in New York City called LISC (the Local Initiatives Support Corporation) that fosters collaborative, community-based, large-scale affordable housing projects. Then she experienced divine intervention: "These two priests came to see me one day and basically said, 'Why can't you do for homeless housing what you've done for affordable housing? We have the solution for housing the homeless mentally ill.'"

The two priests, Franciscan fathers John Felice and John McVean, explained that with some effort they had bought and refurbished first one dilapidated single-room-occupancy hotel near Penn Station and then another. Now they were using them to house and provide health services for people affected by severe mental illness.

Sandorf recounts, "I said to them, 'I don't know anything about homelessness. I don't know anything about mental illness. It's not what we do here at LISC. I'm really sorry, I wish I could help you, but I can't.' I thought I would be damned to Hell because I said this to two priests."

A few months later, Sandorf left LISC to consult on community development for the Pew Charitable Trusts. Realizing that she now had greater resources within her sphere of influence, she decided to go see the priests and their converted hotels, which they had christened St. Francis Residence I and St. Francis Residence II, after St. Francis of Assisi.

"The people who were living there were coming straight out of Bellevue," she recalls. "They were very sick folks."

But they were tenants with leases and private rooms, and they were free to come and go as they pleased. Mainly they came. The priests had persuaded St. Vincent's Hospital to provide staff support to monitor and distribute medicines. Without the medications, the whole thing would have been impossible.

"What we were trying to provide for those people," recalls Father McVean, who along with Father Felice still runs the St. Francis facilities, "is what social workers called—and still call—the activities of daily living. We were helping them with their medication, helping them to get some sort of money, helping them attempt to socialize. Schizophrenia is a very isolating disease, so we had all sorts of activities to try to help them break through that."

While in the city that day, Sandorf visited another building, a housing facility in the Washington Heights neighborhood created by a homeless advocate named Ellen Baxter. Baxter's project was similar to the St. Francis residences, but she catered to a more diverse population and offered a broader array of support services.

Sandorf was "completely blown away," she remembers. "Here were two examples of dignified housing, a place of one's own with a complement of support services designed to support people's independence. And at about half the price per head of what the shelter system was going for. They were putting together these projects with glue and paste, basically, pulling money from here and there but with no organized or systematic way to do what seemed to be the most common-sense solution on earth.

"I said, 'This is the smartest thing I've ever seen. Why isn't this public policy?'"

What she would soon discover while visiting a number of cities on a Pew research grant was that housing with support services was an idea that just seemed to be in the air. Community-based nonprofit organizations in every city she visited were doing some version of it.

"None of these organizations knew about one another," Sandorf says. "They were all sort of figuring it out on their own. There were variations in the kinds of housing, but the fundamental principles were the same. So this was more than some anecdotal success story in New York City.

"They were all doing it by scratching together money from lots of different housing capital programs and then trying fundraising year after year for an array of service dollars, but it was completely disorganized and incredibly painstaking, and every time a new project was done they were reinventing the wheel."

What was needed to take the concept to scale and really make a dent in homelessness, she realized, was an intermediary organization to capture and share expertise, create models and systems that could be replicated, educate public agencies, exploit government funding streams, and provide early capitalization to get projects rolling—sort of a housing-with-services consulting firm with brokerage and banking capabilities. In short, what was needed was the Corporation for Supportive Housing.

Sandorf returned to New York and within three months had raised $10 million in grants to found the organization. The Robert Wood Johnson Foundation put in $4 million. Pew invested $4 million as well. The project represented a departure from the sort of enterprises that typically interested the Ford Foundation, which, through LISC and Enterprise Community Partners had focused on creating affordable housing in distressed communities for people with limited incomes, whether they were homeless or not. But Ford contributed the remaining $2 million. Sandorf remembers one of her colleagues later suggesting that Ford's leadership "was so astounded by my chutzpah that they decided they wanted to participate." She adds, "I had no idea what I was doing, but you have to be young and naïve to think you can do these kinds of things."

After making her pitch to the Robert Wood Johnson Foundation, which is in Princeton, New Jersey, she telephoned her lawyer in New York, whom she would meet shortly to file for nonprofit status. "By the time you get here, you'd better have a name for your organization," he said. She didn't like "service-enriched housing" or "special-needs housing," two descriptions used by some at the time, she says. On the train ride from Princeton to New York she invented "supportive housing," which today is the only term anybody uses.

The Robert Wood Johnson's investment in the Corporation for Supportive Housing now stands at nearly $27 million. After awarding the initial $4 million grant in 1991 to create CSH, the Foundation invested another $4 million three years later to enable the organization to expand to Chicago, Columbus, Ohio, New York City, and the states of Arizona (the program there was discontinued in 1998), California, Connecticut, Michigan, Minnesota, and New Jersey. (The Ford Foundation and Pew Charitable Trusts also continued their support of CSH in 1995). A pair of $6 million grants, in 2002 and 2005, funded a program called Taking Health Care Home, the Foundation's national initiative to help develop a pipeline of supportive housing that could lead, in a single decade, to the creation of the 150,000 units of supportive housing deemed necessary to end chronic homelessness. Another grant—$740,000 awarded in 1995—helped CSH develop an integrated network of more than thirty public agencies and private nonprofit groups to provide an array of needed services to supportive housing projects in California. The resulting supportive housing model established a superior prototype that could be used elsewhere around the country.

The Foundation's most recent grant to CSH, $6 million awarded in February of 2006, seeks to advance CSH's efforts to use supportive housing to help prisoners released from prison—who are not eligible for federal housing subsidies—stabilize their lives and escape the cycle of homelessness, incarceration, and recidivism.

Today the Corporation for Supportive Housing occupies a unique place in the archipelago of social service and community support organizations, not for its unusual smorgasbord of abilities (who else can get you a capitalization loan, a psychiatric social worker, and an instant professional network all for the asking?) but because it is the only organization in the country focused exclusively on the creation of supportive housing for people who are chronically homeless.

"There are organizations similar to ours that have a much broader focus on affordable housing—for *all* people who need affordable housing,"

Carla Javits says. "But the focus that we have on this particular population and on this intervention and the expertise we have in the financing and partnerships and the methodologies for how you do permanent housing with services for the poorest people with the biggest problems—that is unique."

Supportive Housing in Practice: Arnold Stringfellow

Ask Arnold Stringfellow when he moved in to the Camelot Hotel, a supportive housing facility on Turk Street in San Francisco's Tenderloin district, and he responds precisely: "May 11, 2003." Stringfellow has an unusual ability to remember dates and other numbers; more often than not, they are attached to painful memories. He was in the Navy for eleven months and thirteen days. He moved in with his lover on December 31, 1969. He lost his lover to AIDS in 1993, has been in therapy since 1996, lost his home in October of 2002, spent thirty-seven days in a psychiatric institution.

Fifty-seven and lean as a whippet, Stringfellow slicks his hair straight back over his balding head, leaving it longish and curly at the neck. Most of his teeth are missing. He wears a nondescript mustache and a little chin hair on a soft, gentle face that conveys vulnerability. Two keys hang from a black strap around his neck, and he keeps a ballpoint pen in his shirt pocket.

Stringfellow's mother died when he was four. His father worked in a sawmill, planing boards and making pallets, and was married five times. "As far back as I can remember, I've always had thoughts of ending my life," he says. "Because I knew I was different, I couldn't fit in anywhere. I only had one friend when I was little, and one day I saw him get killed on the railroad tracks by a train, and then I didn't have *any* friends."

He was seven years old at the time. His friend's father was racing another car, speeding toward a train crossing. After the collision, Stringfellow ran to his friend, tried to talk to him, watched him die. "I never tried to make any other friends."

The Navy stationed Stringfellow on Treasure Island in San Francisco Bay, where he trained to be a radar man. "I really believed that doctors could make me straight," he says. "So I went to a priest, and after I sat in his office for an hour and a half, I was finally able to tell him what was wrong. He sent me to a psychiatrist, and from there . . ." He lets the sentence hang in the air. "They discharged me with an honorable discharge."

Stringfellow held down a job most of his life. He worked as a temp, an accountant, a computer programmer. He even had his own electronics repair shop for a year and a half. Self-taught, he says. Eventually, though, he found himself broke and on the streets. "I thought I could buy love and affection," he says. "I let people take advantage of me. When the money was gone, they were gone."

He had never imagined himself being homeless. He was fifty-four years old. The first night didn't go well. "Not much sleep. No blanket, no pillow, just a shirt. It was drizzling. I tried to find a piece of cardboard to lie on." The second night, he climbed into some bushes in a futile attempt to stay warm. The nights became months. "Sleeping on the sidewalks was really difficult for me," he says.

With guidance from two psychiatric professionals, Stringfellow found his way to a security shelter, temporary housing and, finally, the Camelot, a narrow, six-story hotel with a clean gray-and-burgundy exterior that stands out among the squalor that surrounds it. One of the ironies you discover upon touring supportive housing projects is that they often tend to be the best-looking buildings on the block, freshly painted and in good repair. The idea is to create a secure, inviting environment where tenants feel safe and have a sense of dignity.

Stringfellow's room on the fifth floor is reminiscent of a room in a well-kept college dorm, small and utilitarian but quite civilized. It contains a sink, a stovetop, a mini-fridge, and a microwave oven (every week he gets seven frozen meals from Project Open Hand and makes one trip to the store for groceries), a narrow platform bed with drawers under it, a chair on casters that he found on the sidewalk, a small closet, a small table, and a telephone that automatically rings the front desk when he picks up the receiver. It also contains electronic equipment, mainly things Stringfellow has found on the street and repaired: a computer, a television, a DVD player, a VCR, a stereo receiver. One wall is exposed red brick, as stylish as a bistro. The floor is covered in a dusty-rose carpet, and a ceiling fan hums overhead. The door has a double lock.

Like most supportive housing tenants, Stringfellow covers a percentage of his rent with his monthly benefit checks. The rest is subsidized. "I love my home," he says. "It's a blessing from God. Every morning, when I get up, I make my bed. At night, I take out my trash. I even polish my sink. I keep it clean and pretty."

Stringfellow is not the typical supportive housing tenant in that he was homeless for months, not years. But he is very typical in that he is afflicted by a combination of physical and mental health problems: attention deficit disorder, depression, high blood pressure. He is HIV-positive. He used to hear voices until doctors put him on the right medications.

The Camelot was created by Direct Access to Housing, an initiative of the Housing and Urban Health unit within the Community Programs Division of the San Francisco Department of Public Health. The facility has an on-site social services manager and a staff of social workers, and every tenant has a case manager to help where help is necessary. The Camelot does not have an on-site medical clinic, but another Direct Access to Housing project nearby, the Windsor Hotel, does, and it serves more than 3,000 supportive housing tenants citywide.

The Direct Access to Housing program has twelve buildings encompassing more than 800 units. The Corporation for Supportive Housing helped make it happen by providing technical and funding guidance. "They're good at both advocating for supportive housing and facilitating the expansion of supportive housing," says Dr. Josh Bamberger, Housing and Urban Health's medical director. "So they're both on the front end and the back end of what we do. They had researchers who were looking at what made the model successful and then got some numbers on paper that we could use as the basis for grant writing for expanding and the basis for testifying to government officials about generating monies. That was critical."

—⚭— Supportive Housing in Retrospect

Julie Sandorf guided CSH from its birth in 1991 until June 1999. Javits, who joined the organization within a year of its inception after working as a legislative analyst for the state of California and then as a social services administrator for San Francisco city government, became the organization's third president and chief executive officer in late 2000.

Javits has short, dark-brown hair with a smidge of gray, brown eyes that twinkle when she is amused, and a hearty laugh. When someone is speaking, she listens hard, often with a slight squint. If she has an affinity for her work, she comes by it honestly. Her father was Jacob Javits, the longtime United States senator from New York. "I grew up with a strong orientation around public policy and social justice," she says. "I was always interested in what could be done to level the playing field for people who are poor and haven't had a fair break in life."

Javits believes that for all its technical expertise, the best and most vital role that CSH plays is "as a convener, bringing parties together to share information and knowledge." Josh Bamberger, the medical director for San Francisco's Housing and Urban Health Unit (see sidebar), singles out that attribute as well. "They are really good at connecting us with other organizations that are doing similar work so we can learn from them and they can learn from us," he says.

No more of the wheel reinventing that Sandorf found so prevalent around the country before she invented CSH. "They're very sophisticated," the Foundation's Nancy Barrand says. "They have depth on their bench. I don't worry about their misstepping or even missing things. They're putting our money to use in a very sophisticated way, using our imprimatur where they need to and in a way that we feel comfortable with. In other words, we trust them to go out and use our money appropriately and wisely.

"But they work in a field where we don't have a lot of contacts. So for them to go out and attract the money of a Deutsche Bank—I wouldn't even know where to start. It's not something that we as a foundation do very well. They allow us to leverage other dollars as well as work with very diverse partners, particularly on the private side. So we get more out of this than just creating supportive housing."

"The Robert Wood Johnson Foundation should get credit not just for seeing that they could move beyond health care and be useful in other ways that are still true to their mission," says Somers, "but also for seeing that they should do it in partnership with other foundations and that they should invest the kind of resources they have invested in it."

Julie Sandorf needed "a couple of years' distance" to fully appreciate what she had set in motion. Having surrendered the CSH reins seven years ago, now she has that perspective. "We absolutely revolutionized public policy with respect to how the public finances and houses the most vulnerable people," she says, taking pains to stipulate that "we" includes all of CSH's funders and partners, especially "the local organizations that had to go through the hell of actually building these deals.

"Supportive housing is now business as usual. That's amazing, given the complicated nature of the work. There are very few times you can look at the social history of public policy over the last several decades and say, 'Something has changed dramatically for the better.' I have a much easier life now, but I know we made history, and that's very thrilling."

Notes

1. Larson L. "Interview with Philip Mangano: Part Two." *Spare Change,* April 4–17, 2002. The full interview was subsequently titled "Hearts and Minds: A Conversation with the Bush Administration's Point Man on Homeless Policy, Philip Mangano" and posted on the Internet at www. realchangenews.org.
2. The estimate for the overall number of homeless is from The Urban Institute analysis of data collected by the U.S. Bureau of the Census in the landmark National Survey of Homeless Assistance Providers and Clients, conducted in 1996. See Burt, M., and Aron, L. Y. *Helping America's Homeless: Emergency Shelter or Affordable Housing.* Washington, D.C.: Urban Institute Press, 2001, pp. 49–50. The estimate for long-term homelessness is from the Partnership to End Long-Term Homelessness, which provided these figures upon announcing its formation in November 2004.
3. Culhane, D. P., Metraux, S., and Hadley, T. "Public Service Reductions Associated with Placement of Homeless Persons with Severe Mental Illness in Supportive Housing." *Housing Policy Debate,* 2002, *13*(1). pp.107–163.
4. Goldman, H. H. "The Program on Chronic Mental Illness." *To Improve Health and Health Care 2000: The Robert Wood Johnson Foundation Anthology.* San Francisco, Jossey-Bass, 1999.
5. Rog, D. J. and Gutman, M. "The Homeless Families Program." *To Improve Health and Health Care 1997: The Robert Wood Johnson Foundation Anthology.* San Francisco: Jossey-Bass, 1997.

7

SPARC—Sickness Prevention Achieved through Regional Collaboration

Paul Brodeur

Editors' Introduction

Every year, the *Anthology* features one chapter that takes a close look at an innovative community-level program and individuals who have worked to improve health locally. The preceding five volumes of the *Anthology* have contained chapters on programs to provide services for homeless pregnant women in San Francisco,[1] prevent violence in crime-ridden Chicago neighborhoods,[2] train inner-city high school and middle school students to run the Los Angeles Marathon,[3] curb alcohol addiction among Native Americans in Gallup, New Mexico,[4] and open a high school exclusively for addicted teenagers in Albuquerque.[5]

This year is no exception. In this chapter, Paul Brodeur, an award-winning former feature writer on health and the environment for *The New Yorker* and a frequent *Anthology* contributor, tells the story of SPARC (Sickness Prevention Achieved Through Regional Collaboration), a program designed to bring preventive health care services to individuals living in the tri-state area of eastern New York, northwestern Connecticut, and southwestern Massachusetts. Largely the creation of physician Douglas Shenson, SPARC provided primary care services in a number of innovative ways, such as its "Vote and Vax" campaign that referred senior citizens for vaccinations as they were approaching or leaving polling places on election day.

The Local Initiative Funding Partners Program, a collaborative effort between the Robert Wood Johnson Foundation and local foundations that supports creative community health efforts, funded the program. The idea behind Local Initiatives is, on the one hand, to leverage the resources and know-how of local foundations and, on the other hand, to develop opportunities for the Robert Wood Johnson Foundation to identify promising ideas that emerge from local leadership and creativity.[6]

1. Diehl, D. "The Homeless Prenatal Program." *To Improve Health and Health Care, Vol. VII: The Robert Wood Johnson Foundation Anthology.* San Francisco: Jossey-Bass, 2004.
2. Diehl, D. "The Chicago Project for Violence Prevention." *To Improve Health and Health Care, Vol. VIII: The Robert Wood Johnson Foundation Anthology.* San Francisco: Jossey-Bass, 2005.
3. Brodeur P. "Students Run LA." *To Improve Health and Health Care, Vol. IX: The Robert Wood Johnson Foundation Anthology.* San Francisco: Jossey-Bass, 2006.
4. Brodeur, P. "Combating Alcohol Abuse in Northwestern New Mexico: Gallup's Fighting Back and Healthy Nations Programs." *To Improve Health and Health Care, Vol. VI: The Robert Wood Johnson Foundation Anthology.* San Francisco: Jossey-Bass, 2003.
5. Diehl, D. "Recovery High School." *To Improve Health and Health Care, Vol. V: The Robert Wood Johnson Foundation Anthology.* San Francisco: Jossey-Bass, 2002.
6. Wielawski, I. M. "The Local Initiative Funding Partners Program." *To Improve Health and Health Care 2000: The Robert Wood Johnson Foundation Anthology.* San Francisco: Jossey-Bass, 1999.

T wo P.M. on a rainy November afternoon at an influenza vaccination clinic in the gymnasium of St. Peter's Parish Center in Great Barrington—a town situated in the southwestern corner of Massachusetts in the foothills of the Berkshires. A dozen or so elderly residents of the town and the vicinity have rolled up their sleeves and lined up before tables staffed by several members of the Berkshire Visiting Nurses Association, who are administering flu shots. It is an activity being carried out at this time of year in flu clinics across the nation, but with one important difference here. In Great Barrington, each woman who has received her flu shot is being asked if she has had her annual mammogram, and if her answer is no, she is being offered an appointment time to get one at either of two regional hospitals. The effort to combine the delivery of flu shots with the making of mammogram appointments is just one of a number of similar preventive health initiatives undertaken during the past ten years by a nonprofit organization called SPARC, which stands for Sickness Prevention Achieved through Regional Collaboration. SPARC acts as a catalyst by bringing local agencies together to coordinate the delivery of preventive care to the inhabitants of four adjoining counties at the intersection of three states—Berkshire County in southwestern Massachusetts, Litchfield County in northwestern Connecticut, and Dutchess and Columbia Counties in eastern upstate New York—which cover an area about twice as big as Rhode Island, and contain some 680,000 residents.

On this afternoon, the SPARC initiative is being overseen by Linda Cormier, a registered nurse who for the past two years has been manager of the organization's rural programs in Berkshire County south of the Massachusetts Turnpike, in the eastern half of Dutchess County, and in all of Litchfield County. White-haired and bespectacled, Cormier has lived in the Berkshires for the past twenty years and is highly familiar with the territory she is responsible for covering. "We use the word 'bundling' to describe the practice of combining one preventive service with another," she explains. "In addition to bundling flu shots with mammograms, other SPARC projects combine flu shots with pneumococcal vaccinations, which guard against the organism that can cause bacterial pneumonia and meningitis, and with cardiovascular disease risk assessments that include tests for cholesterol and blood sugar levels, blood pressure measurement, and education about the hazards associated with smoking and obesity. On election day earlier this month, one of my collaborators went to Clinton, New York, and conducted a cardiovascular risk assessment of voters at a polling center. The people there were thrilled and want us to come back next year."

Cormier goes on to explain that these and various other SPARC projects are being financed by a three-year Rural Health Outreach grant awarded by the U.S. Health Resources and Service Administration's Office of Rural Health Policy. "Unfortunately, this grant will run out in April of 2006," she says. "After that, we'll need to raise additional money to keep our projects operating. In the meantime, we've been partnering with the Centers for Disease Control and Prevention's federally funded program for mammograms and Pap tests to provide early detection of breast and cervical cancer in uninsured and underinsured women. In this regard, it's important to remember that SPARC does not perform any preventive clinical services on its own. We're simply an incubator and facilitator for new ideas in delivering public health care. As such, we depend upon some fifty collaborating agencies either to provide direct patient care, as the visiting nurses are doing by giving flu shots this afternoon, or to help identify and serve new populations of people who are not receiving adequate health care."

In addition to the Centers for Disease Control and Prevention, or CDC, among SPARC's national and state partners and collaborators are the American Cancer Society, the American Lung Association, the Connecticut Department of Public Health, the Massachusetts Department of Public Health, the New York State Department of Health, the Albert Einstein College of Medicine, the AARP, and the Robert Wood Johnson Foundation. Among its Litchfield County collaborators are the Charlotte Hungerford Hospital, the New Milford Hospital, Sharon Hospital, and the Visiting Nurse Services of Connecticut. Among its Dutchess County partners are the Dutchess County Department of Health, the Eastern Dutchess County Rural Health Network, and the Northern Dutchess,

St. Francis, and Vassar Brothers hospitals. Among its collaborators in Berkshire County are the Berkshire Medical Center, the Berkshire Taconic Community Foundation, the Pittsfield Board of Health, and the Berkshire Project HEROA—which stands for Health, Education, Resources, Outreach, and Advocacy.

As it happens, Cormier is being assisted on this particular afternoon by two of SPARC's dedicated collaborators, whom she refers to as the project's "champions." They are Marie Barsousky, who has worked for the New England Division of the American Cancer Society, in Pittsfield, for twenty years, and Lorie Harrington, a registered nurse at the Berkshire Medical Center, who works part-time for Project HEROA, as well as for the Women's Health Network, an organization funded by the Massachusetts Department of Public Health with money provided by the CDC. Cormier and her two colleagues are taking turns approaching women who have just received their flu shots, but their inquiries are almost identical. "I'm here at the flu clinic to help women make appointments for their annual mammograms," they say by way of greeting. "Are you by any chance due for one?"

—⚹— Origins and Early Activities of SPARC

In April of 1994, Michael Alderman, chairman of the Department of Epidemiology and Social Medicine at the Montefiore Medical Center/Albert Einstein College of Medicine, and Douglas Shenson, an internist and assistant professor in the department, published an op-ed piece in the *New York Times* that criticized President Bill Clinton's plan for national health reform, because it overemphasized improved access to physicians while neglecting the importance of delivering clinical services that had proved to prevent disease and extend life. The two physicians wrote as follows:

> Too few people get the vaccinations that prevent infections and the mammograms, Pap smears and examinations that can detect cervical, breast and colon cancers while they are still curable. Nor do most people with high blood pressure or elevated cholesterol receive effective treatment that can prevent strokes and heart attacks. These cancers and cardiovascular diseases together account for half of all deaths in the United States.

Later in their piece, Alderman and Shenson suggested, "Just as local school authorities are responsible for providing primary and secondary education to all, a public health corps built on local health departments could take responsibility for a community's preventive needs."[1]

As things turned out, the ambitious vision of Alderman and Shenson for a public health corps built on local health departments never came to fruition. Instead, as a member of the board of the Berkshire Taconic Community Foundation (an organization established to pool the philanthropic resources of the residents of Berkshire, Litchfield, Dutchess, and Columbia Counties), Alderman persuaded his fellow board members to take on the prevention of disease as a critical task for the foundation. Virgil Stucker, who was then director of the foundation, proceeded to convene several meetings of regional residents and visiting experts—among them local hospital officials, physicians, visiting nurses, and directors of rotary clubs and senior centers—to consider how the foundation might become involved in the delivery of preventive health care. In June of 1994, the board voted to award a $10,000 grant for the planning and initial development of a preventive disease program—a task that was taken up by Shenson, who became the program's executive director, and whose services were initially made available by the Albert Einstein College of Medicine. Soon afterward, to further this effort, an anonymous board member of the foundation made a $20,000 challenge grant that was quickly matched by local residents.

By the spring of 1995, SPARC—an acronym devised by Shenson, who then thought up the words to fit it (Sickness Prevention Achieved through Regional Collaboration)—had begun to develop along several lines. First and most challenging was the task of raising funds for operating costs; second was the need for developing projects that would carry out SPARC's mission of expanding the delivery of disease prevention services; and third was the necessity for establishing an independent governance structure. The last of these was accomplished through Michael Alderman's efforts. He recruited an independent board of directors, that, in turn, led the way for SPARC, originally a creature of the Berkshire Taconic Community Foundation, to become an independent not-for-profit corporation.

During the next several years, program development came to be the province of half a dozen steering committees, which grew out of the meetings initially convened by the Berkshire Taconic Community Foundation's Virgil Stucker, and whose members assumed responsibility for delivering clinical preventive services in their own localities. The number of steering committees increased until, by the beginning of 1997, they partly covered Berkshire and Dutchess Counties and were operating in all of the communities in Litchfield County.

From the beginning, the steering committees included preventive health providers, as well as other private, public, and nonprofit partners, who not only were knowledgeable about the preventive health care needs of their respective localities but also possessed expertise in delivering it. The first of them, which was formed in Lakeville, Connecticut, met in the summer of 1995. Among its members were representatives of a local hospital, the visiting nurse association, the Older Women's League, the mental health association, and two local physicians. They adopted the overall SPARC program for delivering clinical preventive services, which, as defined by the United States Public Health Service, include influenza vaccination; pneumococcal vaccination; childhood immunizations; adolescent immunizations; mammography; Pap smear; test for fecal occult blood; sigmoidoscopy or colonoscopy; blood pressure measurement; and cholesterol measurement. Of these services, influenza vaccination for the elderly was identified as the most appropriate and important first step by the members of the Lakeville group, as well as by each of the other steering committees.

A major contribution to the early development of SPARC was the concept advanced by Shenson that the various components of clinical preventive services should not only be delivered separately to patients by physicians practicing primary care medicine, as had been the case in the past, but should also be considered as a unified endeavor, and, whenever possible, be administered in combination. Influenza and pneumonia shots had previously been combined at a number of locations across the nation, but in 1996 Shenson came up with the novel idea of bundling flu and pneumonia shots with appointments for mammograms. The experiment, supported by a grant from the Patrick and Catherine Weldon Donaghue

Medical Research Foundation, was first tried in Litchfield County the following year, and led to a doubling of mammography use there. As a result, the flu-mammography project has since become one of SPARC's major initiatives.

Other SPARC efforts to increase provider and recipient participation in preventive care were implemented early on by the organization's steering committees. For example, the Northern Berkshire County Committee sent flu shot reminder letters to all individuals over the age of sixty-five who resided in one of its pilot sites. Additional pilot sites for the delivery of clinical preventive services were established in the modest-income town of North Adams; in a poor urban neighborhood on the west side of Pittsfield; and in the semi-rural town of Great Barrington. Medicare reimbursement records for Litchfield County indicate that since the inception of SPARC's influenza vaccine initiative, in 1995, the county had risen from third place in the delivery of flu shots to elders to the top rank among Connecticut's eight counties.

—ᴡᴡ— The Role of the Robert Wood Johnson Foundation

During its first two years, the SPARC program raised $180,000 from foundations and nongovernmental organizations interested in supporting pilot disease prevention projects. During that same period, private philanthropy provided SPARC with more than $100,000, demonstrating the commitment of local residents to improving the health of their communities. However, if SPARC were to achieve its ambitious goal of furnishing clinical preventive services to all the residents of its four-county area, it was obvious that more resources would be required. Consequently, in December of 1996, Shenson undertook to write a grant proposal to the Local Initiative Funding Partners program of the Robert Wood Johnson Foundation. He was assisted in this endeavor by Virgil Stucker and by Donna DiMartino, a community nurse specialist at Sharon Hospital, who had been lent to SPARC by the hospital, which also paid her salary.

Thanks largely to the vision of Terrance Keenan, then a senior program officer at the Foundation, the Local Initiative Funding Partners program had been created in 1987 to encourage partnerships with smaller foundations that, like the Robert Wood Johnson Foundation, fund projects in the area of health and health care. Local Initiative Funding Partners is a program of matching grants designed to support collaborative relationships between the Robert Wood Johnson Foundation and local foundations that finance innovative community-based projects to serve people who are underserved and at risk. Robert Wood Johnson Foundation grants averaging between $200,000 and $500,000 per project are paid out over a three-to-four-year period and are awarded through a competitive process. The philosophy guiding the Local Initiative Funding Partners program is that local grant makers interested in addressing local health care problems have a knowledge of their communities that no national foundation can match.

As it happened, the Local Initiatives Funding Partners program had turned down two previous requests for funding submitted by Shenson. However, staff members there had been sufficiently impressed by SPARC's mission and early accomplishments to encourage Shenson to keep applying, with the understanding that SPARC would be required to raise local funds to match any grant awarded by the Local Initiative Funding Partners program.

In his December 1996 proposal for funding, Shenson declared, "Despite their extraordinary benefits to health, national data indicate that the use of clinical preventive services is well below the accepted targets of *Healthy People 2000*."[2] (This publication of the U.S. Department of Health and Human Services set goals for improving the public's health.) He also wrote, "A major reason that clinical preventive service rates are low in the United States is that no defined public or private body takes responsibility for assuring that all residents in a community are presented with an informed choice and reasonable access to these services." In this regard, he indicated that SPARC would address such fundamental problems "by developing a program that takes responsibility for increasing access to clinical preventive services for *all* residents in the region." The proposal further indicated that SPARC would promote at least seven of the ten clinical preventive services in 50 percent of the Berkshire-Taconic region within four years and that in those communities served by the program, the gap between current utilization rates and an ideal rate of 100 percent would be reduced by half.

To carry out these ambitious goals, Shenson presented the Local Initiative Funding Partners program with a list of planned activities. Among them were the expansion of an adolescent health project in Berkshire County, under which arrangements had already been made with two high schools to vaccinate adolescents born before 1994, when hepatitis B immunization became mandatory for newborns. In the grant application, Shenson proposed extending the hepatitis B initiative into high schools in West Side Pittsfield and Poughkeepsie, followed by expansion into Hudson, New York, and rural towns in Columbia and Dutchess Counties. Among other initiatives in the proposal were the expansion of early cancer detection projects to increase women's access to mammograms and Pap tests, investigating whether flu clinics could successfully serve as places to connect older women with breast cancer screening, increasing influenza and pneumococcal vaccinations among the elderly, and developing an information system to guide and evaluate efforts to increase access to clinical preventive services.

Persuaded by SPARC's goals and by the plan for reaching them, the Robert Wood Johnson Foundation, acting on the recommendation of the staff of the Local Initiative Funding Partners program, awarded the Berkshire Taconic Community Foundation a matching grant of $425,000 to be used by SPARC over a four-year period commencing on August 1, 1997 and ending on July 31, 2001. Financial support from the Robert Wood Johnson Foundation's Local Initiative Funding Partners program was a critical milestone in the continuing development of SPARC. The award received wide local publicity, earned SPARC credibility with collaborators and members of the community, and provided fiscal stability to a financially fragile organization. During the next few years, donations from small foundations and local contributors combined to match the Local Initiative grant, and a series of "at home" meetings provided an opportunity to familiarize small groups of invited guests with the program and to broaden its base of support.

Another important source of funding for SPARC was contracts with the agencies in Massachusetts, Connecticut, and New York that monitor the quality of services delivered to Medicare beneficiaries. These contracts made it possible to offer individual preventive services, such as flu and pneumococcal vaccinations and referrals for cancer screening. They also were important because the agencies' reimbursement records helped determine whether the SPARC projects were improving the delivery of preventive health care.

Over the next four years, SPARC made significant strides in increasing the delivery of clinical preventive care to residents of the four-county area. By the end of the grant's second year, the organization had established steering committees across the entire Berkshire-Taconic region, and assured access to flu shots for elderly residents in all communities of the four counties. This represented an outreach to approximately 95,000 residents age sixty-five and older. In addition, SPARC made access to pneumococcal immunizations possible for some 80,000 elderly residents of Berkshire, Dutchess, and Litchfield Counties, and expanded its initial mammography-flu project across all of Litchfield County and part of Dutchess County. The project reached out to some 2,000 women age fifty and older, and in a three-month period served 338 women who had not received a mammogram in the previous year. Finally, SPARC's school-based hepatitis B vaccination program grew 140 percent in the first two years, and reached 1,560 adolescents.

During the third year of the Local Initiative grant, SPARC continued to make progress as influenza and pneumococcal immunizations were made available at all public clinics in the Berkshire-Taconic region. SPARC's innovative approach to mammography—the bundling of flu shots with appointments for screening for breast cancer—was expanded to all of Litchfield and Dutchess Counties. SPARC's hepatitis B immunization project expanded from serving three schools in Litchfield County to serving seven schools in Litchfield and Columbia Counties. In Dutchess County, SPARC launched a new initiative to promote screening for colorectal cancer.

In the fourth and final year of the grant, public clinics in the SPARC service area reported a 15 percent increase in influenza vaccinations and a 21 percent increase in pneumococcal immunizations. The organization broke new ground by launching an initiative promoting screening for diabetes, hypertension, and breast cancer among residents of the African-American and Hispanic communities of Poughkeepsie and Beacon, New York. SPARC also expanded its flu-mammography initiative and undertook a pilot replication of the project in Ulster County, on the west side of the Hudson River. For the first time, however, geographic expansion was not the propelling force behind SPARC's program development. Instead, new emphasis was placed on building links with physicians and creating networks of practice-based nurses to extend the use of immunizations and cancer screening among patients.

—៳— Further Development of SPARC

In testimony before the House Subcommittee on Oversight and Investigation on May 23, 2002, David Fleming, a physician who was then the acting director of the Centers for Disease Control and Prevention, declared that the SPARC approach to preventive services was worthy of national replication. "The SPARC model has demonstrated its value in bringing lifesaving preventive services to older adults," Fleming said. "Communities around the country could benefit from innovative and successful models like SPARC."[3]

As it happened, staff members of the Robert Wood Johnson Foundation were already interested in replicating the SPARC initiative, and the Foundation's Local Initiative Funding Partners program had recently awarded SPARC a one-year grant of $25,000 to assess its impact on the regional delivery of preventive care, and to disseminate the results in the medical literature in order to facilitate replication of the SPARC program. The assessment, which is ongoing, is being conducted by SPARC in collaboration with the Yale-Griffin Prevention Research Center, in Derby, Connecticut. The dissemination of its results has been undertaken by Shenson, who has been writing and publishing articles about SPARC's history and accomplishments and about the potential role that the SPARC program can play in expanding preventive care services.

Testifying before the Special Committee on Aging of the United States Senate, on May 19, 2003, James S. Marks, then the director of the CDC's National Center for Chronic Disease Prevention and Health Promotion and currently a senior vice president at the Robert Wood Johnson Foundation, said that "SPARC has demonstrated great success in enhancing the provision of preventive services within clinical practices, facilitating public access to prevention, and establishing local account-ability for the delivery of services." Later in his testimony, he declared that the organization "represents a particularly noteworthy catalyst for enabling an effective community-based response to a national priority."

Meanwhile, the U.S. Government Accountability Office, which is concerned with the cost-effectiveness of government programs, had turned to SPARC for advice on how to improve Medicare's delivery of preventive services; the Massachusetts, Connecticut, and New York departments of health had asked SPARC for help in developing replica-ble disease prevention initiatives; and officials of CDC's National Immu-nization Program had sought SPARC's response to potential changes in national immunization policy. The immunization program's interest in SPARC was not surprising. In the autumn of 2002, the organization had completed a five-year hepatitis B vaccination program during which nearly 2,000 adolescents were immunized.

During 2003, funds provided by the CDC enabled SPARC to con-tinue expanding the delivery of flu shots and pneumonia vaccines to the residents of the Berkshire-Taconic region. As part of this effort, the orga-nization placed advertisements in newspapers urging people to get flu shots, and arranged for public service announcements on major radio stations. Funding from the CDC and from the Massachusetts Medicare quality improvement agency, MassPRO, enabled SPARC to establish networks of practice-based nurses in communities in Berkshire and Litch-field Counties, with the expectation that such networks would extend the use of mammograms, cholesterol screening, pneumococcal immu-nizations, and fecal occult blood testing. Using funds obtained from the Dyson Foundation, SPARC developed a team of trained commu-nity members, called peer health advisers, to identify persons at risk for diabetes, hypertension, or breast cancer in the hard-to-reach populations of the African-American and Latino communities of Poughkeepsie and Beacon. With funds from the Pfizer Foundation, and in collaborations with the Yale-Griffin Prevention Research Center, SPARC convened and conducted a series of focus groups made of up of African-Americans with diabetes in order to inform them about diabetes control and proper foot care. This initiative developed into a formal research project that evaluated the impact of a tailored brochure designed to improve foot care among diabetic African-American patients.

When a pilot project called Homebound Adults identified 128 Meals-on-Wheels recipients in Berkshire County as needing flu shots, and five recipients who needed pneumococcal vaccinations, SPARC hired visiting nurses to provide the appropriate immunizations.[4] With these findings in mind, the leaders of SPARC made several key recommendations to the Connecticut Department of Public Health to ensure that the vulnerable population of homebound adults in that state would not go without flu and pneumococcal immunizations. As a result, the department provided SPARC with funds to expand its Homebound Adults initiative to Litchfield County. In addition, SPARC developed a project called Prevention Sundays to increase adult immunizations and cardiovascular screenings in rural eastern Columbia County. In this project, SPARC collaborated with the Columbia County Department of Health and the Columbia County Community Healthcare Consortium to promote, coordinate, and implement four church-based clinics offering members of their congregations and the public at large cholesterol screenings, as well as tetanus, diptheria, and pneumococcal immunizations. Funding for Prevention Sundays was provided by the Our Town Fund, the Berkshire Taconic Community Foundation, and the Hudson River Bank & Trust Foundation.[5]

—⁂— The Federal Rural Health Outreach Grant

In the spring of 2003, the Office of Rural Health Policy of the U.S. Health Resources and Services Administration awarded SPARC a three-year $196,000 outreach grant to ensure that long-standing programs, such as adult immunizations, would emphasize initiatives that served hard-to-reach populations in isolated rural areas. One goal of the Rural Health Outreach Grant Program was to increase the delivery of annual influenza vaccinations to people fifty and older by 10 percent, and to increase the delivery of pneumococcal vaccine to people sixty-five and older by 20 percent. In order to accomplish these objectives, SPARC and its collaborators undertook to:

- Develop a calendar/flyer listing the locations of public flu clinics, and the dates and times they would be open.

- Establish and maintain a twenty-four-hour flu clinic information hot line to provide callers with the same information.

- Coordinate the schedules and the distribution of the clinics to provide maximum accessibility.

- Place announcements about the availability of flu shots and other preventive services on local television and radio programs, and in newspapers and posters.

- Send physicians in the target area material explaining the initiative and encouraging them to immunize their patients when appropriate.

A second objective of the outreach project was to achieve a biannual mammography rate of 80 percent in women aged fifty and older who were participating in the immunization clinics program, and a colorectal screening rate of 50 percent among men and women aged fifty and older who were participating in the program. Women of fifty and older would be asked if they had had a mammogram within the past twelve months, and, if not, would be offered the opportunity to receive a scheduling call from a radiology facility of their choice. Men and women of fifty and older who had been identified as overdue for colorectal cancer screening would be asked permission for SPARC to send a letter to their physician informing them that such screening might be in order.[6]

In the autumn of 2003, SPARC conducted a survey called Prescription for Life at thirty-two community flu clinics to determine whether the respondents had received timely immunizations and cancer screenings. The survey was completed by 2,025 participants, of whom 1,375 were women. Three hundred and sixty of these women stated that they had not had a mammogram in the previous twelve months; 145 of them requested mammogram appointments; and sixty-seven of them received mammograms within the next eight months. The importance of the Prescription for Life initiative was soon apparent. Two of the sixty-seven mammograms showed abnormalities, and both of the women involved were found to have developed breast cancer.

During the three-year period of the rural health outreach grant, SPARC maintained its activities in the African-American and Latino communities of Dutchess County, and continued working with the CDC to help health care and civic leaders in other regions develop the skills to launch their own SPARC replication sites. Among the minimum requirements for such sites were the ability to assess local baseline delivery rates for clinical preventive services; a history of successful collaborative activities; the presence of a lead agency that could function as a neutral convener of clinical preventive services' providers; the ability to involve all sectors of the local health care delivery system, such as hospitals, public health organizations, and medical practices; the ability to combine or bundle clinical preventive services' delivery; and the capacity to evaluate the result of the intervention. In this last regard, SPARC declared that it would promote the publication of outcomes data from its own work and from that of the replication sites—the idea being that a critical mass of evidence would be needed to confirm the hypothesis that creating accountable agencies for the communitywide delivery of clinical preventive services could lead to measurable increases in the delivery of such interventions.[7]

SPARC's Vote and Vaccinate Project

In the spring of 2004, Shenson was invited to attend a Local Initiative storytelling skills workshop held at the Robert Wood Johnson Foundation. The story he told was how, in 1997, after learning about an idea that had been tried in the South—offering flu shots to elders after they had voted at polling places—Donna DiMartino, the nurse specialist at Sharon Hospital, and some of her nursing colleagues decided that such an activity might make a worthwhile project for SPARC. However, they soon discovered an old Connecticut ordinance that prohibited commercial activities of any kind near a polling station. Fortunately, with the assistance of a state representative, who happened to sit on one of SPARC's steering committees, DiMartino was invited to testify before a committee of the Connecticut Legislature. Impressed by her testimony emphasizing that more than any other group, older people show up at the polls on Election Day, which happens to fall right in the middle of the flu shot season, the committee instructed the state attorney general to review the law with an eye to permitting flu clinics to operate near polling places. As a result, in 1998, SPARC piloted a clinic for voters in the town of Salisbury, Connecticut, which proved so successful that in the following year Vote and Vax clinics, as they came to be called, were established across Litchfield County, and have since become part of the way flu shots are administered in all of the communities in which SPARC is active.

Based on the results of SPARC's Vote and Vax initiative, in September of 2004, the Robert Wood Johnson Foundation awarded fifteen health departments across the nation grants of up to $8,000 each to help local communities organize and implement influenza vaccination clinics for low-income and hard-to-reach adults over the age of fifty at or near polling places on Election Day, 2004. A major goal of the program was to increase the number of flu shots to elderly African-Americans and Hispanics, who were lagging far behind whites in vaccination rates. The Foundation also authorized a grant of $58,000 from the Local Initiative Funding Partners program's special opportunity fund to enable SPARC to develop criteria for eligibility and selection of grantees and provide technical assistance to them.

The 2004 Vote and Vax Project was assembled at a very quick pace. By August 2, completed applications from sixty prospective grantees had been submitted, and by the end of the month fifteen health districts from across the nation had been awarded funding for the initiative. However, in mid-September, Chiron, one of the two U.S. flu shot manufacturers, announced that it was having production problems, and in early October it ceased production altogether, leaving ten grantees with a shortfall of vaccine. Members of the project steering committee decided that those grantees unable to provide flu shots would not be asked to return their funds but would be asked instead to develop public health outreach or provide other vaccinations at clinics near polling places. In the end, twelve grantees launched activities at fifty-six polling stations, where they delivered a total of 1,030 flu shots, 224 pneumonia shots, 91 tetanus shots, 70 hepatitis A shots, and 52 hepatitis B shots.[8]

Virtually all of the health departments that received grants saw Vote and Vax as a public health opportunity to be exploited, and voter reaction was overwhelmingly enthusiastic. Most important, the fact that every grantee was able to work with local election authorities to establish a Vote and Vax clinic demonstrated that the establishment of such clinics on Election Day was replicable. As a result, Vote and Vax was now considered to be in a position to be used as a model around the nation.

With this in mind, the Foundation issued a report in the early autumn of 2005, entitled *Vote and Vax: Setting up a Successful Clinic in Your Community.*[9] The report pointed out that on November 8, 2005, more than 100 million Americans would come together to vote at their local community polling places, that approximately half of them would be fifty years old or older, and that making flu shots available at clinics convenient to polling places might significantly reduce the 20,000 deaths that occur annually in the United States as a result of influenza. It recommended that the leaders of Vote and Vax projects consult with local election officials to make sure that their activities conformed to local or state law, and it urged them to consider that the middle of the day—between 10 A.M. and 5 P.M.—might be the period during which large numbers of elderly voters would come to polling places. In May, 2006, the Robert Wood Johnson Foundation awarded SPARC a grant of $321,000 to expand Vote and Vax to twenty-five additional low-income communities across the nation in anticipation of the November 2006 elections and flu season.

—w— SPARC's Founders Talk about Its Future

Michael Alderman is an unassuming, gray-haired man in his late sixties, who has been chairman of the board of SPARC since the organization's inception. In addition to being instrumental in the founding of SPARC, he has provided extraordinary leadership in helping to formulate strategic objectives for the organization, and in sharing his expertise as one of the nation's leading epidemiologists. "I've been wondering if a non-profit organization such as SPARC is the ideal model for replication nationwide," he said in a recent interview. "My concern is, why go to the expense and trouble of creating yet another structure when we might be able to do without it? Perhaps the most efficient way to provide clinical preventive services might be through consortiums of hospitals—say, two to five hospitals in a given region—that would work together and form their own steering committees in order to come up with their own ideas about how to deliver clinical preventive services."

Alderman went on to say that he had already been exploring this idea with Sharon Hospital, Fairview Hospital, and the Berkshire Medical Center. "The role of SPARC would be to share with the hospitals our familiarity with the local communities in the region, and thus help make them become more efficient in the delivery of preventive services," he explained. "Hopefully, SPARC might also be able to raise money for the consortiums from outside organizations, such as Medicare and the CDC, which have already invested in SPARC projects. Hospitals invariably want to make connections with people in the communities they serve. For that reason, delivering immunizations, cardiovascular screening and cancer screening would make for excellent public relations, not to mention increased profits. Right now, the greatest challenge for SPARC is sustainability—how to raise sufficient money to keep providing and expanding the delivery of clinical preventive services in our four-county area."

Alderman's continuing interest in the delivery of clinical preventive services on a large scale was on display a few weeks later on November 30, 2005, when he published an op-ed piece in the *New York Times,* which advocated treating people who might become afflicted with avian flu with the vaccine effective against the pneumococcal bacteria that causes pneumonia. According to Alderman, such treatment might save the lives of up to 25 percent of those infected with influenza, because patients weakened by the disease often acquire bacterial pneumonia. In addition, Alderman called for a government program to guarantee life-saving vaccines for every American. "Such a program would replace our shamefully inadequate and unfair private system of vaccine delivery," he wrote. Alderman ended his piece by declaring that the kind of program he was recommending not only would improve survival in a future natural or man-made catastrophe but also "will put in place the means for regular delivery of all the tools—not just vaccines—that prevent disease and safeguard our health."[10]

Douglas Shenson is a soft-spoken, forty-nine-year-old man who was born in England of American parents and came to the United States to attend boarding school, in 1970. Later, he completed a joint program in medicine and public health at the Tulane University School of Medicine, in New Orleans, and a residency in internal medicine at the Montefiore Medical Center, in the Bronx. While at Montefiore, he worked with AIDS patients in the inner-city population, which opened his eyes to the need for preventive services throughout the nation.

After describing how SPARC has significantly raised the rates for vaccinations and cancer screening among the residents of the Berkshire-Taconic region, Shenson went on to say that a major reason for this achievement has been that, from the beginning, the organization never tried to compete for the delivery of preventive health services. "That would have made partnerships more difficult to establish," he explains. "Instead, we have striven to create alliances with these providers and to collaborate with them to increase the delivery of clinical preventive services. In this way, by acting as a bridge between medicine and public health, SPARC has built a whole new approach to prevention that considers physician practices as simply one element in a communitywide network of activities."

Over the past two years, Shenson has worked with colleagues at the CDC to analyze data on the delivery of clinical preventive services. The results of this work highlight the magnitude of the problem SPARC is trying to address. "About 95 percent of adults aged sixty-five and older have health insurance through Medicare, which pays for cancer screening and vaccinations," Shenson points out. "However, fewer than 40 percent of this age group are up to date with basic preventive services, such as immunization for influenza and pneumonia, and screening for breast, cervical, and colorectal cancers. And when you include the younger group—adults aged fifty and older—who should be receiving these services, fewer than 27 percent are up to date on all of them. One reason for this is that most physicians are accountable only for the patients in their practices. Nobody has taken responsibility for the prevention of disease in the community as a whole."

Like his colleague Michael Alderman, Shenson has been thinking long and hard about how to create an effective nationwide program that might emulate the achievements of SPARC. "How do you develop a system with local accountability for the delivery of potentially lifesaving preventive measures when there is currently no such system?" he asks. "In my opinion, the question begs for an experiment that will evaluate the ability of a variety of agencies and institutions to serve as potential platforms for replication of the SPARC program. Among the candidates are consortiums of hospitals, local or state public health agencies, academic medical centers, and organizations that deal with the nation's aging population. It seems to me that of all the ways we have of investing our money in preventive health, such an experiment is both necessary and promising. Let's hope that the nation's public health officials will be able to muster up the vision and determination to carry it out."

—ᗯ— SPARC's Program Manager Assesses Her Efforts

Four P.M. at the flu/mammography clinic in St. Peter's Parish Center in Great Barrington. Linda Cormier and her two colleagues are talking to the last of several women who have received flu shots before the clinic closed. Afterward, she reveals the results of the afternoon. "Most of the two dozen women we queried today had already received mammograms within the past twelve months," she says. "However, four women who had not received a mammogram—among them a mother and daughter—made appointments to have them at Fairview Hospital. All in all, I consider that a wonderful response to our effort here."

Cormier goes on to describe the continuing need for clinical preventive services in the Berkshire-Taconic region. "A large part of our population is subject to seasonal layoffs," she points out. "Among them are people who work as waiters, waitresses, and kitchen help in bed and breakfast establishments, inns, and restaurants, as well as farmers, agricultural workers, carpenters, roofers, snow plowers, and people working in the ski industry. Such people are often uninsured or grossly underinsured. There's also a great need to take the flu/mammography project to special groups of women—factory workers, health care workers in hospitals and nursing homes, schoolteachers, school bus drivers, and other women who work part time. Women school bus drivers could be canvassed at their annual safety meetings, or as they wait for children to be let out of school. The mothers of school children could be approached on parents' night. As you can tell, I'm a great believer in the flu/mammography project, and feel that it should be taken nationwide. It's easy to carry out, it's inexpensive, and, most compelling of all, it saves women's lives."

—◁◁◁— Conclusion

On December 12, 2005, SPARC received the Aetna Susan B. Anthony Award for Excellence in Research on Older Women and Public Health. This award is given annually by Aetna and the Gerontological Health Section of the American Public Health Association, or APHA, to honor individuals whose research has made significant differences in the lives of older women. It specifically recognized the value of SPARC's innovative flu/mammography project, and was received on behalf of SPARC by Linda Cormier at the American Public Health Association's annual meeting in Philadelphia.

The APHA award to SPARC is a public recognition of the program's accomplishments in increasing the delivery of clinical preventive services to the residents of the Berkshire-Taconic region during the past ten years.

Not the least of SPARC's accomplishments is the fact that many of its projects, such as its flu/mammography initiative and the Vote and Vax project, have been demonstrated to be replicable. The time has now come for major governmental health agencies at the state and federal level to determine how best to replicate a SPARC-like program nationwide that will spread the delivery of immunizations and cancer screening to a vast population of people who are without them at present and therefore are at avoidably greater risk of developing potentially fatal diseases.

Notes

1. Alderman, M., and Shenson, D. "A Ton of Cure." *New York Times,* April 24, 1994, op-ed page.
2. National Center for Health Statistics. *Healthy People 2000 Final Review.* Hyattsville, Maryland: Public Health Service. 2001 (http://www.cdc.gov /nchs/data/hp2000/hp2k01.pdf)
3. SPARC. *SPARC Annual Report,* June 2002, cover text.
4. Ibid. pp. 2–9.
5. SPARC. *SPARC Annual Report,* 2003–2004, pp. 7–9.
6. Ibid. pp. 12–17.
7. Ibid. p. 18.
8. Shenson, D. *Vote and Vax Project Report.* Prepared for the Robert Wood Johnson Foundation and the Local Initiatives Funding Partners program. April 6, 2005, pp. 2–10.
9. The Robert Wood Johnson Foundation. *Vote and Vax: Setting Up a Successful Clinic in Your Community.* (http://www.rwjf.org/files /newsroom/votevax091405.pdf)
10. Alderman, M. "The Flu's Second Front." *New York Times,* November 30, 2005, op-ed page.

8

The Southern Rural Access Program

Digby Diehl

Editors' Introduction

The most consistent priority of the Robert Wood Johnson Foundation, dating back to its earliest days, has been to expand access to medical care for underserved individuals, a disproportionate number of whom live in rural areas. Although 20 percent of the U.S. population lives in rural areas, only 9 percent of America's physicians work there. Because the 60 million people living in rural areas tend to earn less than people living in or near cities, health problems associated with poverty, such as infant mortality and many chronic diseases, are often more serious in rural areas.

The federal government is the key player in attempting to improve health care services in rural areas. Its efforts include the Health Resources and Services Administration's rural health and community health centers; the Indian Health Service's programs, which are largely, but not only, rural; and the National Health Service Corps, which forgives loans made to physicians and other health professionals practicing in underserved areas. State governments, too, have developed programs to attract health care professionals to rural areas.

The Robert Wood Johnson Foundation has employed a number of approaches to improve health services for people living in rural areas. The Practice Sights program, for example, supported states' efforts to attract health care professionals to rural areas.[1] The Reach Out program encouraged physicians to volunteer their services to people living in underserved areas, many of which were rural.[2] A variety of efforts provided training of and encouragement to nurses, nurse practitioners, and physician assistants practicing in rural areas.[3] The Foundation has provided scholarships to medical students from rural areas (on the assumption that they were likely to return to practice there), promoted rural hospitals, and developed rural perinatal care networks and rural physician group practices.

In this chapter, the award-winning author and frequent *Anthology* contributor Digby Diehl looks at a program designed to improve access to medical care for people living in some of the nation's most underserved areas—the rural South of the United States. The Southern Rural Access Program addressed some of the most important barriers that keep physicians from locating in rural areas of Alabama, Arkansas, Georgia, Louisiana, Mississippi, South Carolina, East Texas, and West Virginia. In this chapter, Diehl chronicles the ways in which the grantees went about attracting health care professionals to rural practice and the many challenges they faced, including the devastation wrought by Hurricanes Katrina and Rita. Even after the program ended in 2006, the infrastructure that it had established in Louisiana and Mississippi provided a foundation for some of the post-hurricane reconstruction efforts.

1. Wielawski, I. M. "Practice Sights: State Primary Care and Development Strategies." *To Improve Health and Health Care, Vol. VI: The Robert Wood Johnson Foundation Anthology.* San Francisco: Jossey-Bass, 2003.
2. Wielawski, I. M. "Reach Out: Physicians' Initiative to Expand Care to Underserved Americans." *To Improve Health and Health Care 1997: The Robert Wood Johnson Foundation Anthology.* San Francisco: Jossey-Bass, 1997.
3. Keenan, T. "Support of Nurse Practitioners and Physician Assistants." *To Improve Health and Health Care 1998–1999: The Robert Wood Johnson Foundation Anthology.* San Francisco: Jossey-Bass, 1998.

—ᴡ—**A**ll grant making entails a leap of faith, but launching the Southern Rural Access Program required more leaps—and more faith—than most. The project began with the faith to allow a Robert Wood Johnson Foundation program officer, Michael Beachler, to pursue his strong belief that the Foundation should undertake a rigorous effort to improve health care in the dramatically underserved areas of the rural United States. The Foundation board made another leap of faith when it deviated from long-standing policy and identified the specific eight medically needy states the program would fund without knowing which agencies would lead their states' efforts.

In a considerable departure from standard procedure, the Robert Wood Johnson Foundation convened workshops in each recipient state so that key stakeholders could confer and agree on a lead nonprofit agency for the Southern Rural Access Program. After that lead agency had been identified, the Foundation provided financial and technical assistance to help the lead agency write grant applications to the Foundation. Finally, after the grants had been awarded, the leaders in each state made decisions about investments and techniques of intervention for particular regions within broad strategic components monitored by the Access Program's national program office. The grants were of varying size and duration. Once the program was launched, each state progressed at its own pace and followed its own agenda. All recipients were faced with significant challenges, the most tragic of which were the double devastations of Hurricanes Katrina and Rita, which ripped through many of the participating Southern Rural Access Program states.

Because the Southern Rural Access Program has only recently concluded (in March 2006) at a total cost of $36 million, including a revolving loan fund and 21st Century Challenge Fund grants, not enough time has passed to be able to gauge its long-term impact. It is not yet possible to determine how successful the Southern Rural Access Program will be in sustaining the grant-funded programs, though the early evidence is promising in most of the eight states. From the outset, some states were better organized than others, and therefore made more significant progress. Even those states that struggled initially, however, have implemented most aspects of the program's agenda. It is also too soon to know whether successful Southern Rural Access Program interventions and techniques will eventually be replicable in other rural areas. Nonetheless, even given this limited perspective, the Southern Rural Access Program has clearly produced some major beneficial effects. Steps have been taken to create and strengthen regional health infrastructure; revolving loan projects and philanthropic partnerships are continuing in most of the states; and the problems of rural health access have a higher profile with both federal and state agencies throughout the Southern Rural Access Program areas.

—ɯ— How the Program Was Formulated

"I recall seeing Michael Beachler in the workout room of the Foundation," says Steven Schroeder, former president of the Robert Wood Johnson Foundation. "He would be sweating copiously, pounding on those machines with a ferocity that was unmatched by anyone else. You could hear the machines groaning. That is the same level of energy and dedication that Beachler brought to developing a program for rural health care." Beachler had been recruited to work for the Foundation in 1987 and immediately plunged into Healthy Futures: A Program to Improve Maternal and Infant Care in the South. In 1991, he turned his attentions to Practice Sights: State Primary Care Development Strategies, which attempted to bring a variety of primary medical services to underserved areas of the United States.[1]

"At the end of most Robert Wood Johnson programs, the program officers are asked to present 'lessons learned' at a staff meeting, and I talked about some of the positive aspects of the Practice Sights Program and some of the things that didn't work quite as well," Beachler recalls. "This sparked a discussion within the staff about how the Foundation had not been entirely successful in coping with the areas of poorest health care, primarily in rural areas. After consultation with Dr. Schroeder, I was tasked to design a program based on several of the Foundation's rural investments, but one that would be more comprehensive in its approach to the problems of the underserved communities. I tried to incorporate ideas from my experiences with Healthy Futures and Practice Sights, as well as other Foundation work, such as the Hospital-Based Rural Health Care Program."

Eventually, many of these previously tested interventions were combined with new ideas to make up the four primary components of the Southern Rural Access Program:

- *Recruitment and retention* of medical personnel in rural areas.

- *Revolving loan funds* to finance primary health care and other health care facilities in rural areas.

- *Rural health networks* to provide a multicounty or multiparish infrastructure for mutual support and economy of scale.

- The creation and support of *rural health leaders* who come from involved communities.

An additional component emerged from discussions with other philanthropies:

- *The 21st Century Challenge Fund,* a matching grants program much like the Local Initiative Funding Partners previously established at the Foundation.

Beachler's initial proposal, created over the subsequent six months, embraced what he called the Rural Axis—a large geographic area comprising up to sixteen states that included not just the South but the Dakotas, Wyoming, and Montana as well. An effort of this size was deemed unrealistic by other staff members, so Beachler and others began the process of narrowing the geographic scope of the program. Nancy Kaufman, then a Robert Wood Johnson Foundation vice president, recalls, "We created national maps with various overlays for poverty, infant mortality, access to health care, and other indices. The rural South consistently had the worst problems in the country, so we felt that we had to focus on that area." More than 40 percent of all Americans in persistent poverty live in the South.[2]

One statistic generated by Foundation staff research was particularly persuasive in the decision to concentrate on the South. An internal review of Foundation investments between 1992 and 1996 compared spending in Minnesota with spending in five of the most underserved Southern states: Mississippi, Louisiana, South Carolina, Alabama, and West Virginia. According to an article in the *Journal of Rural Health,* "The 'Needy Five' have roughly 3 times as many residents, 7 times as many uninsured and poor people, and 17 times as many residents living in shortage areas [as compared to] Minnesota." However those five states combined received only 76 percent of the funding awards made by the Foundation to Minnesota in that same period.[3]

As contiguous states with similar health problems, Arkansas and Georgia were subsequently added to the Needy Five. Using the same reasoning, Kaufman argued forcefully for the inclusion of Texas in the program. "The reason I felt so strongly was that I could see border issues, immigration problems, and other new health problems arising in that state," she recalls. "There was also very strong health leadership in Texas at that time. I felt that we could get ahead of the curve." Although Schroeder objected that adding such a large state was too ambitious for a pilot program, a review of the statistics pointed the way to a middle ground. When Kaufman, Beachler, and other staff members looked at demographics and key health issues, they discovered that East Texas statistically resembled the rest of the South far more than it did the rest of Texas itself. As a result, just East Texas was added to the program as the last of the Southern Rural Access Program states.

⟋⟍⟍⟋ The Beginnings of the Southern Rural Access Program

"One key moment was a meeting that the Foundation convened in February of 1997," Beachler recalls. "It was held in New Orleans, just before Mardi Gras, and we brought representatives from fourteen Southern and Great Plains states to discuss the general idea of the Southern Rural Access Program project. We batted around the concepts that were starting to jell within the Foundation, and asked for opinions. The Southern Rural Access Program was unanimously well received by the constituents from those states."

In July of that year, the Foundation's board authorized $14.5 million for a broad range of initial grants, technical assistance, and planning to implement the Southern Rural Access Program in eight states over three years. Included was $800,000 to establish a national program office at the Penn State College of Medicine in Hershey, Pennsylvania, with Beachler as director and Isaiah Lineberry as deputy director. Floyd Morris, who was then a program officer at the Foundation, worked closely with Beachler and Kaufman in conceptualizing the Southern Rural Access Program, and made the presentation of the project to the board. "When I presented the proposal to the board, I explained how we needed to be flexible and develop a program that would respond to the long-term needs of these rural underserved Southern states," Morris says. "I also emphasized the fact that if we were going to make lasting changes to the rural health care infrastructure in the South, we needed to stick with it for a long time."

The Robert Wood Johnson Foundation board was very supportive. "I think they were very much aware that this part of the country was underrepresented," Schroeder recalls. "As a whole, they felt that the management strategies we had devised were reasonable, granted that there were risks."

At the inception of the program, one question arose consistently: Why is a program for eight Southern states headquartered in Hershey, Pennsylvania? As Beachler points out, there are actually three answers to that question. First, when the location for the national office was selected, it was envisioned that the program would cover a large portion of the United States; under that assumption, Hershey seemed as reasonable as anywhere else. Second, Beachler had strong relationships with many colleagues at the Penn State College of Medicine who had experience in rural health care. Third, and perhaps most important, the Foundation initially planned to work with a large integrated rural health delivery system that was being formed in 1997 through the merger of the Geisinger Health System, the Penn State College of Medicine, and the Milton S. Hershey Medical Center (the merger was dissolved two years later).

The national program office officially opened on October 1, 1997, with two major tasks: to staff and start up the office and to inform the individual states about the program. Achieving the latter task involved a considerable divergence from standard Foundation policy. Traditionally, a single applicant workshop was held in a central location. For the Southern Rural Access Program, however, the board approved allocations to hold eight separate applicant workshops, one in each state. The intention was to permit each state to identify its own lead agency and to allow Foundation staff members to advise that agency on grant-writing procedures. Other state stakeholders, including local philanthropies, banks, hospitals, health care providers, economic development agencies, and local United States Department of Agriculture staff, were invited as a way of making the entire regional community aware of the Southern Rural Access Program. Beachler recalls that six of the states quickly identified a lead agency, often through the state Office of Rural Health. Alabama and Mississippi deliberated for two or three months before focusing on an agency.

In yet another departure from Foundation policy, each state was given $15,000 to fund planning meetings for the preparation of grant proposals. In traditional grant-making procedure, grant applications are received within six to eight weeks after the workshop. The Southern Rural Access Program allowed much greater flexibility, so that the start-up time for each grantee was longer. The first Southern Rural Access Program grant was awarded to the South Carolina Office of Rural Health in December of 1998.

—₥— The Program in Three States

South Carolina

"When the Southern Rural Access Program came along, I had been on staff in the South Carolina Office of Rural Health for a while, and I felt as though our state was already doing pretty well with some of the things the Foundation was suggesting," recalls Graham Adams, executive director of the Office of Rural Health. "We were better organized than many states to take advantage of the program, and there is no doubt that the Southern Rural Access Program enhanced and strengthened the programs we had already begun. However, we were a little slow to see the big picture of networking and infrastructure that Beachler kept hammering at us. The greatest gift that the Southern Rural Access Program gave us was the ability to understand how to make all of the necessary elements work together to create a synergy."

The South Carolina Office of Rural Health was established as an independent 501(c)(3) nonprofit organization in 1991, so it was almost immediately recognized as the natural lead agency in that state. At the time the Southern Rural Access Program was initiated, the Office of Rural Health was already overseeing several successful programs. Its Rural Health Revolving Loan Program was set up in 1997 with a $900,000 Rural Business Enterprise grant from the United States Department of Agriculture. A program to provide vacation relief for rural doctors, which had emerged from the University of South Carolina in 1994, became a key element of the Southern Rural Access Program medical recruitment and retention efforts. The Southern Rural Access Program also facilitated the expansion of an existing South Carolina Rural Interdisciplinary Program of Training. A new Community Incentive for Diversity program was designed to encourage minority nurse practitioners, physician assistants, and certified nurse midwives to go into underserved rural areas.

The first grant was for a fifteen-month planning and pilot implementation period. The Robert Wood Johnson Foundation allocated $458,000 to establish elements of the Southern Rural Access Program in a seventeen-county region in the eastern part of the state, which encompassed nearly 664,000 people. "To begin, there was a lot of complaining and criticism about the four core elements of the Southern Rural Access Program," says Amy Brock Martin, who began as a coordinator and quickly became director of the Southern Rural Access Program in South Carolina. "The public health mantra is that the community should identify the problem and drive the solution. For that reason, many people resisted a foundation that pushed us to focus on these four elements. I think, in retrospect, I can safely say that they were wrong. I credit Michael Beachler, this courageous Yankee who came down here and helped us use our own creativity to meet this model, but insisted that we include these four principles. I don't think we all understood how interconnected these principles were until we began to implement them. Frankly, it was really brilliant."

Mitch Wilkins, the revolving loan specialist for the South Carolina Rural Health Access Program, recalls that the existing revolving loan program really took off with an infusion of both capital and prestige from the Robert Wood Johnson Foundation. "We marketed the program with a series of conferences throughout the state, and it just mushroomed through word of mouth," he says. "Wachovia Corporation has become our largest partner, although we work also with community banks. Probably 75 percent of our loans go through commercial banks. This is a perfect project for banks to meet the requirements of the Community Reinvestment Act, and our work ranges from doing the underwriting and legwork for the loan right up to being a fifty-fifty partner in some of the medical start-ups. One of the most impressive facts about our program, from the viewpoint of the financial community, is that we have never had a single default since we began." Since the inception of the program, the South Carolina revolving loan program has facilitated 111 loans totaling more than $43 million.

"We use a lot of different resources to attract physicians into our rural communities," notes Mark Griffin, the director of recruitment for the Office of Rural Health. "This is a small state with a good highway system, and we are pocketed with hospitals in both urban and rural areas—we have half a dozen large ones. The vast majority of the recruitment I do is through the hospitals, because they can guarantee doctors a salary until they are ready to step out into their own practices. Then Mitch can help them with the financial issues and Marsha Marze, our rural health clinic coordinator, provides technical support for their practice management. Our state is also a great retirement area, so we have an impressive supply of older experienced doctors who are wonderful part-time primary care physicians or *locum tenens* substitutes."

Locum tenens is a Latin term that describes a physician who temporarily takes over the practice of another doctor. South Carolina's *locum tenens* program now covers the entire state, and is divided into three regions, each of which has a set of doctors ready to step in to provide relief to colleagues seeking a vacation, further medical education, or just a little time off from stressful work. Griffin's office coordinated roughly 320 weeks of *locum* relief in the first year.

The *locum tenens* program is particularly important in areas where there may be only one family practitioner or obstetrician in the community. In the town of Bamberg (population 3,700), for example, the Michael Watson Rural Health Clinic serves a patient base that includes impoverished African Americans, a nearby Mennonite community, and a seasonally shifting group of Hispanic migrant farm workers. "The South Carolina Department of Health mandates that the obstetrician on call may never be more than thirty minutes away from his hospital to be available for emergency caesarean sections," says Laura Hoffman, Watson Clinic office manager. This is a reasonable requirement, except that William Glenn, director of the Watson Clinic, is the only obstetrician in Bamberg County. Not surprisingly, after several years of being continuously on call, he began to feel burned out. "The poor man was tethered to Bamberg for years without a break," Hoffman continues. "When he did take a vacation, we had to hire both an OB and a family practice physician to substitute for him, and the expense was impossible. Now, with the *locum tenens* program, he can have a life and our clinic has good quality substitutes at a reasonable cost."

Just across the street from the Watson Clinic, near the Bamberg County Hospital complex, are the modest offices of the Low Country Health Care Network. Cathy Schwarting, executive director of the network, points out, "Before the Southern Rural Access Program, we never entertained the idea of networking, sharing ideas, health problems, and sometimes solutions. The four county hospitals in the four counties that I represent—Bamberg, Allendale, Barnwell, and Hampton—certainly did not cooperate before we started meeting with them. They saw each other as competitors. Now they share a radiology group that services all four hospitals. Through the revolving loan program, the network purchased a mobile MRI unit that travels to each hospital on different days of the week on a regular schedule. They are all linked by PACS, a computer accounting system that allows them to communicate about patients. We are now looking into converting all of our hospitals into one hospital information system that will make available medical records of all patients in the area. The Southern Rural Access Program allowed us to have the time and the manpower to brainstorm and discover common ground. The state offices are now setting up two other networks—one in the Fairfield area and one in Newbury. Health networking is a concept that is here to stay in South Carolina."

Schwarting is a graduate of the South Carolina Rural Interdisciplinary Program of Training, or SCRIPT, which is a five-week rural immersion program for health profession college students. The program, directed by Diane Kennedy, provides an opportunity for students to actually work in rural areas and experience rural life. "Many of the students have come from rural areas and are already inclined to return," Kennedy says. "Others see the advantages of small town life, particularly when raising a family. And then there are always a few who can't stand the quiet or the lack of movie theaters. That's okay too, because there is no point in trying to recruit people who are already disinclined." Initially funded by the Southern Rural Access Program, the SCRIPT program is continuing with grants from local, state, and federal resources. By the end of 2005, it had graduated a total of 609 students from six participating universities.

Similarly, the Community Incentive for Diversity project provides scholarship, leadership, and mentoring opportunities for South Carolina minority students in the seventeen Southern Rural Access Program counties. "I never would have been able to complete the nurse practitioner program at the University of South Carolina without the Community Incentive for Diversity project," Wilicia Gaymon says. "Now I am working in a community health center in Eastover, the town where I grew up. I am happy to be near my family and proud to be serving my community."

Two practice management technical assistance programs fostered by the Southern Rural Access Program will also continue in South Carolina. The South Carolina Medical Association operates Project Stay Put, a service that helps private physicians stay financially viable, and the Office of Rural Health has a service that helps facilities that are designated as rural health clinics. Because areas of poverty and poor health care were targeted, fifty-nine of the 105 rural health clinics in South Carolina are in the original seventeen-county Southern Rural Access Program focus area. "We support the existing rural health clinics with billing, coding, and handling the mazes of Medicare and Medicaid, which is how a majority of their patients can afford medical help," says Marsha Marze, coordinator of the clinic program. "We also teach them how to meet the state Department of Health requirements and to be sure that they are compliant with HIPAA [the Health Insurance Portability and Accountability Act of 1996] and OSHA [the Occupational Safety & Health Administration] regulations. We also encourage new clinics. Right now I have eleven providers who are applying for rural health clinic status. Adding them will greatly enhance health care in our poorest areas."

Of the four 21st Century Challenge Fund grants in South Carolina, perhaps the most innovative is the Health and Faith Communities Collaborative Project. Designed to educate people in rural communities about health issues, the program reached deep into the African American communities through their churches. "The initiative took the information to the faith community—the most primary institution in the African American community," says Mary I. Mack, former director of the project. "Through our faith-based initiatives, we were able to reach most of the people in these communities."

Arkansas

The Robert Wood Johnson Foundation board approved the first Southern Rural Access Program for Arkansas on February 1, 1999. The lead agency, a newly formed organization called the Arkansas Center for Health Improvement, received a total of $537,000. Dr. Kate Stewart heads the agency, and at her offices in the Fay W. Boozman College of Public Health at the University of Arkansas for Medical Science, she looked out over a vista of downtown Little Rock and recalled the beginnings of the Arkansas Rural Access Program. "One of the things we struggled with up front was the Foundation's insistence on a prescribed program with four components," she says. "There was already a lot going on in the health area in Arkansas, and we didn't want to duplicate those efforts. As a result, our strategy was to build capacity and to strengthen existing programs, which ultimately has been great for our ability to sustain those programs as the Southern Rural Access Program winds down."

One element already in place was a revolving loan program through the Southern Financial Partners, a nonprofit affiliate of Southern Bancorp, the largest rural development holding company in the United States. "Although we had been in operation since 1986 to help the poverty situation in Arkansas, we had never made any loans in the health care area," says Paul Shuffield, community development officer for Southern Financial Partners. "We were the first revolving loan organization to be granted $500,000 in seed capital by Robert Wood Johnson in October of 1999. We received another $500,000 grant in 2002, and have had generous grants and loans from several other state, federal, and philanthropic sources—most notably the Walton Family Foundation."

By the end of 2005, Southern Financial Partners had leveraged that seed capital into approximately $16 million in health care loans. "We've done everything from cash flow loans for individual providers to financing the construction of hospitals," Shuffield says. "Our first loan was $25,000 to a nurse-midwife to help her get her clinic started. We've made equipment loans to general practitioners and clinics, and built or renovated hospital facilities. You should see the new $4 million 25,000-square-foot health and wellness center that the loan fund financed to house the Delta Area Health Education Center in Helena."

Helena, Arkansas is a sad portrait in poverty. "You are in the highest concentration of rural poverty in America right here," says Mary Olson of the Tri County Rural Health Network Board. A raft of poverty surveys confirm that she is correct—the Arkansas Delta has the lowest income levels and the highest unemployment of all of the rural United States. Olson's office is a storefront on one of the main streets in Helena, a dismal, trash-strewn, empty avenue. There are only two restaurants and a couple of dingy bars. Naomi Cottoms, director of the Southern Rural Access Program's Community Connecting Program, corroborates Olson's bleak overview of Helena: "Our unemployment rate is double that of the state as a whole. Our per-capita income is less than half the national average. Our population is two-thirds African

American. But you don't need statistics. Just look around. There are no jobs."

The Community Connecting Program is a grassroots organization funded by the Southern Rural Access Program through the Tri County Rural Health Network. Cottoms and her five community connectors go door-to-door in the three counties—Lee, Monroe, and Phillips—to link up citizens with health care services. They serve a population of approximately 45,000, spread out over a wide geographic area.

"In this community, health care does not have a high priority, because people are so concerned about food, clothing, and shelter," Cottoms points out. "Many of the people we contact have never had health services in their lives. We connect about 2,000 people each year to a doctor, a dentist, a clinic, or a hospital, most of them for the first time." They also help sick and elderly people to find a way to navigate the tangle of government health bureaucracies that will pay for their care and treatment.

In the Helena Regional Medical Complex, situated away from the bleak downtown area, a more hopeful picture emerges. The Pillow Clinic is run by Dr. John Pillow—and his extended family. His brothers and their wives will eventually all be working here. "Helena is our hometown, and before we went to medical school we knew that we wanted to come back here to raise our families, so we all took advantage of the Community Match Program," says Pillow, speaking in the tiny area that serves both as a lunchroom and a nurse's office.

The Community Match Program pays 50 percent of a medical student's tuition in return for a commitment to work in a designated rural community. "There are nine doctors in the area, so we're able to rotate," Pillow says. "Each of us takes the responsibility of a week on call for the regional hospital every ninth week. Here in the clinic, my brother Gil and I are very busy. We see thirty-five to forty-five patients per day, and our nurse practitioner probably sees twenty to thirty patients. But I love it. I love the town and the people. As a physician, I also like the diversity of pathology that I deal with in a family practice—I see a much more challenging array of problems than I would ever see as a specialist. I'd just like to have a little more time with my family and . . ." he adds, looking around the crowded little lunchroom, ". . . more space."

Joyce Shepherd, who worked with the Southern Rural Access Program recruiting health care providers into the Delta for five years, understands how rare the dedication of someone such as John Pillow can be. "I was born in Wynne, here in the Delta, and after I went to Tulane to work on my master's degree in public health, I swore I would never come back," she says. "But here I am, and I would rather be here than any place else on earth. My recruiting experience is that the financial incentive programs work fine to bring physicians into rural communities, but they really have to be happy in order to stay. More often than not, this means someone who was born in a rural community."

Larry Braden, a physician who came from Hawaii to work in the rural Arkansas community of Camden, agrees. Braden now mentors medical students interested in practicing in rural areas. "I tell my students about the satisfaction I get from primary care medicine in a rural community," he says. "Some of them get it, and some of them are simply headed for brain surgery. More than anything, I think we have to persuade students to ignore the stigma that some medical school professors place on family practice."

Perhaps the most impressive aspect of Arkansas's Southern Rural Access Program experience is the creation of three health care networks—the Arkansas River Valley Rural Health Cooperative, the Delta Hills Community Access Program, and the Crittenden Community Health Council. This trio of agencies began forging links among health care providers so they could pool their resources in practice management, finances, and transportation.

M. Robert Redford, the executive director of the Arkansas River Valley Rural Health Cooperative, created a highly effective two-year demonstration program. His community-based managed health care plan cost less than half the Medicaid average, and provided health care services to a large number of low-income families. "We started in a three-county area with 51,000 people. Now we're going into a new phase with 245,000 people," Redford says. "What excites me is that this model works for the doctors; it works for the hospitals; it works for the patients; and most of all, it works for the state of Arkansas. It is a win-win formula for patching the hole in Arkansas' health care safety net."

Louisiana

Even before the hurricanes, Louisiana was plagued by institutional and political infighting. The beginning of Louisiana's Southern Rural Access Program was delayed by a power struggle between the Louisiana Department of Health and Hospitals and the Louisiana State University Health Sciences Center over which entity would be the designated the Southern Rural Access Program lead agency. Dr. Mervin Trail, the dynamic chancellor of the LSU Health Sciences Center, finally won the turf tussle, but the battle made Louisiana the next-to-last state to receive an initial Southern Rural Access Program implementation grant. It also left a key partner, the Department of Health and Hospitals, with ruffled feathers. After Louisiana received a grant of $513,678 on March 1, 1999, the project director, Marcia Broussard, brought the program up to speed. Together with Ruth Landis, her program coordinator, the two also began to heal the rift between the two agencies.

"The decision to focus the Southern Rural Access Program on the pilot area of southwest Louisiana was not mine, but it was a good one," Broussard recalls. "This is not only an area of tremendous health care need but also of cultural integrity. Historically, it is Cajun country, where the French Canadians settled. We needed a strategy to work on the development of health capacity in communities—and that cultural unity helped us." Broussard identified the closest element to network infrastructure that Louisiana had working for it: the Area Health Education Centers, which began in the 1970s as a national network of community agencies.

"The centers were originally designed to connect the residents in large urban medical schools with rural areas and to provide local health education," explains Jeanne Solis, the executive director of the Southwest Louisiana Area Health Education Center. "We're kind of matchmakers between the urban folks and the rural folks. We're very systems-oriented. There are five divisions in my center: the largest is wellness education; second is recruitment and medical staffing; the third is community health network development; fourth is career education for medical students; and fifth is clinical support services. As you can see, this is very similar to the four core elements of the Southern Rural Access Program, so we were a good match."

The Southwest Louisiana center was contracted to establish pilot programs in networking and recruitment and retention for the Southern Rural Access Program. The development director, Kristy Nichols, was the first employee hired. "We started by doing a survey in the parishes to identify local needs," Nichols recalls. "It was called Health Access Barriers in the South—HABITS—and truthfully it did not discover any problems of health access that were not well known to us anecdotally. It did, however, provide hard evidence of community needs in areas such as medication access, transportation, and financing the uninsured—we were able to quantify the problems. The survey also allowed us to point out that there were eighty-two people in one particular small town who said they needed another doctor in the community. This put a human face on the problem and gave us the voice of the constituents, so that legislators and others in power had to listen."

Nichols began in St. Mary Parish, one of the poorest areas of Southwest Louisiana, and worked with a fledging project called ByNet (the Bayou Teche Community Health Network) to meet the needs identified in the HABITS survey. ByNet implemented a patient assistance program to help individuals get prescription drugs at little or no cost. It solicited donations of medical equipment—hospital beds, canes, crutches, etc.—to be given to needy patients. ByNet also established a medical transportation network through local churches to help patients get to appointments with their physicians. According to the newly appointed ByNet executive director Craig Mathews, the organization is now in the process of establishing relationships with providers within its three-parish area—St. Mary, Iberia, and Terrebonne—to access mental health services.

The second major component of the Louisiana Rural Health Access Program is its revolving loan fund program, headed by Brian Jakes, who is also the chief executive officer of Southeast Louisiana Area Health Education Center. "We were slow coming out of the chute," Jakes recalls. "As a guy who has spent twenty-eight years in the business of banking, it didn't take me long to size up the problem: Louisiana is not a state with a lot of resources for capital formation. We started with two large banks with a strong regional presence and were not successful in working with the home offices. They were cut and dried, not real compassionate. We found it much easier to go into rural communities and establish a relationship with the local bank."

Jakes, a sophisticated banker and stylishly elegant dresser, clearly has a bit of riverboat gambler in his soul. "I made a conscious decision *not* to ask the Robert Wood Johnson Foundation for the initial seed capital," he says. "It was important to prove that Louisiana could get this started on its own." Jakes approached Jim Parks, president and chief executive officer of the Louisiana Public Facilities Authority, which is described as a quasi-governmental public/private funding enterprise, and came away with a $500,000 no-interest loan as seed capital. "At this point, Robert Wood Johnson said that it would match that sum if we could come up with another $300,000," Jakes recalls with a smile. "Well, we went back to Jim at Public Facilities. While we were waiting our turn, their board approved a $60 million bond transaction in about twelve minutes. I said to myself, '$300,000 is going to be a piece of cake!'"

Not exactly—an hour and a half's worth of sweating and grilling later, Jakes came away with the rest of his seed money. He hasn't looked back since. The project has secured additional seed capital from the United States Department of Agriculture ($99,900) and anticipates a $1.2 million award from the Department of the Treasury's Community Development Financial Institutions Fund by early 2007. The Louisiana Rural Health Loan Program has already closed thirty-five loans worth more than $52 million, and expects to have completed $6 million more in loans by the end of 2006.

Almost all of these loans have been made in partnership with small local banks. "There is gratification in working with community bankers," notes Richard Blouin, Jakes' senior loan coordinator. "They know what having a health care provider in a small rural community really means."

The Louisiana Rural Health Access Program was looking strong and sustainable until August 29, 2005. On that day, one of the largest and deadliest hurricanes ever to hit the United States swept in, leaving more than 1,800 people dead. Hurricane Katrina devastated large sections of the Gulf Coast, including areas of Louisiana, Mississippi, Alabama, and 80 percent of the city of New Orleans. Damage is estimated at more than $100 billion. Less than a month later, Hurricane Rita hit Mississippi, Louisiana, Texas, and Arkansas, and added to the misery and devastation that many of these areas had already suffered.

One of the inadequately reported stories of these hurricane tragedies is the great response of outlying areas, especially in southern Louisiana, that were overwhelmed by hundreds of thousands of evacuees from New Orleans and other coastal cities. "All across the state, evacuees were walking into hospitals and clinics with no medical records, no medications, and in need of help," Marcia Broussard recalls. "Our rural coalitions were amazing in their response to health problems, in setting up shelters, in locating food, and many other things. We had a fledging pharmacy access program and some other elements, but what made everything work was network connections. Our offices in New Orleans were gone, but we were able to communicate with our networks of rural providers by cell phone." Michael Beachler adds, "The ability of Louisiana's Rural Health Access Program to respond to the Katrina tragedy was an important demonstration of its value."

—ᴡᴡ— Highlights from Programs in Other States

In carrying out the required elements of the Southern Rural Access Program, the states adopted a variety of approaches. Some highlights:

Recruitment and Retention

Among the most creative programs to address problems of recruitment and retention is West Virginia's Recruitable Community project, which reversed traditional recruitment techniques. Instead of seeking out physicians willing to practice in rural communities, this program, administered by the West Virginia University School of Medicine and the West Virginia Department of Health & Human Resources, works with rural communities to make their towns more appealing to health care professionals who might settle there. Initially, seven communities recruited a total of twenty-seven providers by using this technique. A second, more traditional, program, Coordinated Placement, engaged placement counselors in all three of the state's medical schools—the West Virginia University School of Medicine, the West Virginia School of Osteopathic Medicine, and the Marshall University's Joan C. Edwards School of Medicine. By working together with traditional recruitment techniques, this program continues to place approximately twenty-five health professionals in rural areas every year.

Strengthening practice management formed a part of all states' programs. For example, in East Texas, the Piney Woods Area Health Education Center coordinates the work of the Practice Management Technical Assistance program, which serves forty-two clinics, physicians, and hospitals in the Southern Rural Access Program area, and provides clinics and workshops on billing and coding for family practice residents. At present, this assistance program serves sixteen counties with almost 500,000 people.

Rural Health Networks

Rural health networking figured prominently in the Texas program. The East Texas Health Access Network now serves a five-county area—Jasper, Newton, Sabine, San Augustine, and Tyler counties. It was awarded a federal three-year Health Resources and Services Administration grant for $595,000. The Access Network has expanded its prescription assistance program to 315 medically indigent patients and provides over $1 million in free medications per year.

The Philanthropic Collaborative for a Healthy Georgia funded nine multicultural health networks. A $500,000 Robert Wood Johnson Foundation 21st Century Challenge Fund grant was matched with a $500,000 grant from the Robert W. Woodruff Foundation. The Georgia Department of Community Health then added two grants totaling $1.5 million. Working through the nine separate networks, the Southern Rural Access Program served thousands of impoverished residents in need of health care. The program provided individual case management, mobile screening units, free prescriptions, and programs targeting diabetes, obesity, and cancer. Six of the original nine networks continued at the conclusion of the Robert Wood Johnson funding.

Smile Alabama!, a dentistry program, was jump-started by a $250,000 21st Century Challenge Fund grant. This sum was quadrupled by matching grants from nine other institutions, including the federal government (Medicaid), the Alabama Department of Public Health, and the Alabama Power Foundation. Smile Alabama! increased the number of dentists willing to accept Medicaid by 57 percent; increased the number of Medicaid-eligible children receiving dental treatment by nearly 9 percent; and decreased the number of Alabama counties with no Medicaid dental care from nineteen to ten.

Rural Health Leadership

The East Texas program excelled in the growth and development of new rural health professionals. Described by Michael Beachler as "one of our stronger leadership programs," the Health Career Admission Planning Service, housed at the Piney Woods Area Health Education Center, is a three-tiered program for health care professional students from Texas colleges and universities. Beginning with larger programs and health career convocations, the program provides students who already have an interest in rural health with workshops, and eventually with one-on-one career mentoring.

In Alabama, the Southern Rural Access Program enhanced and connected two rural health leaders pipeline programs. In 1994, the Tuskegee Area Health Education Center had begun a program to make high school students aware of health issues in rural areas. The purpose was to prepare participants for college-level study in the health sciences and eventually for careers in rural health. Under the Southern Rural Access Program, this program was enlarged with specific emphasis on minority students and students from eighteen counties in Alabama's Black Belt.[4] Students received a $1,200 stipend to attend the summer program. This program is now connected to the Rural Medical Scholars program, which originated in 1996 at the Department of Community and Rural Medicine at the University of Alabama Medical School in Tuscaloosa.

Revolving Loan Funds

"Undoubtedly the most stunning achievement of the West Virginia Southern Rural Access Program program is its revolving loan fund," Michael Beachler notes. With an initial Robert Wood Johnson grant of $500,000—later doubled—the West Virginia Rural Health Infrastructure Loan Fund raised a total of $6.97 million in seed capital. This enabled the program to make thirty leveraged loans totaling $15.3 million, funding a wide range of health care projects, including staff augmentation, the construction of new health care facilities, and substantially enhanced service to rural communities.

The Mississippi revolving loan fund is described by Beachler as "the sleeping giant of the Southern Rural Access Program loan funds." Working with the Enterprise Corporation of the Delta, the original $605,000 in Robert Wood Johnson seed capital was leveraged with $3,645,000 to close seven loans totaling $4.25 million by fall of 2005.

—᙮— The Southern Regional Health Consortium

One of the most visible legacies of the Southern Rural Access Program is an interstate group called the Southern Regional Health Consortium, made up of representatives from the eight Southern Rural Access Program states that will continue to meet and exchange ideas. This sixteen-member board (two people from each state), chaired by Steven R. Shelton of East Texas, will continue to share information and discuss regional problems they have in common. "The consortium developed from discussions with Michael Beachler and Anne Weiss at the Foundation about what the legacy of the Southern Rural Access Program might be," South Carolina's Graham Adams recalls. "We seem to be learning a lot from one another, and we have explored different ways to employ the four components of the Southern Rural Access Program program. As a result, we agreed to set up this virtual organization to continue networking." The Robert Wood Johnson Foundation awarded a $600,000 grant to support the concept. Curtis Holloman, former deputy director of the Southern Rural Access

Program, has recently signed a contract to become the project director of the Health Consortium.

Dr. Kate Stewart, head of the Arkansas Center for Health Improvement, was instrumental in the formation of the consortium, which is still in its infancy. She reports that in its earliest meetings the board had agreed to focus on three areas of discussion and cooperation:

■ *Obesity and lack of physical activity*—a particularly acute issue in the region.

■ *Racial and ethnic health disparities*—an exploration of why people of different backgrounds have different health outcomes from the same treatment.

■ *Loan funding for health care.*

Graham Adams adds a provocative note: "I think the Foundation is taking a leap of faith here, as it did with the initial funding of the Southern Rural Access Program. Some of the discussions we have had about the root causes of health problems in our states go way beyond health care. We are talking about racism, education, lifestyle, socioeconomic status, politics, and other elements that affect health. I believe that the work we have begun with the consortium has the potential to be some of the most important work I've done in my career."

—⁓— **Final Grantee Meeting: Lessons Learned**

There is Michael Beachler, out there on the dance floor at the Hilton Lafayette in Lafayette, Louisiana, sweating and stomping in "Don't Mess with Texas" socks and T-shirt, dancing every dance, Mardi Gras beads around his neck, swinging to the infectious washboard beat of Jamie Bergeron and the Kickin' Cajuns. This charming Irishman with his insistent, energetic style has been the driving force of the Southern Rural Access Program from the beginning. He is surrounded by 200 people, most of whom have shared the seven-year journey of the Southern Rural Access Program and have gathered here in February, 2006, for one last time to review what they have learned or accomplished—and to celebrate the finale, Louisiana-style.

A broad extrapolation of thoughts expressed by numerous speakers and panelists at the conference (amplified by notes from a "Lessons Learned" presentation by Beachler on March 9, 2006) suggests the following precepts, organized according to the components of the Southern Rural Access Program:

Revolving Loan Funds—These were vital and successful elements of the Southern Rural Access Program for most of the states, having generated 100 loans totaling approximately $131 million, which is more than an 18:1 ratio to the Robert Wood Johnson investment of $7 million in grants. The key to success was finding a blend of state, federal, and philanthropic resources to provide seed capital. Because of leveraging, all of the loan funds proved to be a more efficient use of public dollars than state grants to individual providers.

Regional Health Networks—Virtually all conference participants agreed on the value of this program element. Economies of scale made providers more efficient, and shared practice management techniques improved revenues. Connecting consumers to multiple available services was more effective than leaving them to find their ways through the medical mazes. Synergies were created between regions, and sometimes between states, through networking. Several participants emphasized the need to generate network revenue through fees or to develop state support.

Recruitment and Retention—Don Pathman of the University of North Carolina at Chapel Hill, director of the evaluation team, noted that the Southern Rural Access Program had achieved the goal of increasing the number of primary care physicians in the target regions. He did, however, raise a troubling question: Did this actually improve health services to the consumer? Beachler pointed out that 114 new providers had been recruited in Mississippi. He also praised the innovative *locum tenens* project in South Carolina. Several participants noted that practice management technical assistance was one of the most effective tools for health provider retention.

Health Leaders—This was generally agreed to be the least effective element of the Southern Rural Access Program. The limited scale of most programs and the lack of support from some schools hindered development. Beachler praised the Community Incentive for Diversity and the Interdisciplinary Program of Training in South Carolina as innovations, and noted the reduced federal spending for a wide variety of health professional programs, which suggests the need for finding other support.

As the evening was winding down in Lafayette, the Robert Wood Johnson Foundation senior program officer Anne Weiss looked out over the festive scene and mused out loud, "I've been to a number of these final grantee meetings. They mark the end of our official involvement in a national program, so even though there is usually a lot to celebrate, there are goodbyes to say too and a certain poignancy to the occasion. You might expect it to feel a little bit more like a funeral, but the food and the music and the laughter at this one are amazing."

Overhearing her remark, Brian Jakes commented, "Didn't you know that all our funerals end like this in Louisiana?"

Notes

1. Wielawski, I. M. "Practice Sights: State Primary Care Development Strategies." *To Improve Health and Health Care, Vol. VI: The Robert Wood Johnson Foundation Anthology.* San Francisco: Jossey-Bass, 2003.
2. MacGregor A. and Warren, D. *Philanthropy in the Rural South: A State Description and Analysis of Assets and Grants.* Raleigh, N.C.: Southern Rural Development Initiative, 2003, p. 463.
3. Beachler, M., Holloman, C., and Herman, J. "Southern Rural Access Program: An Overview." *The Journal of Rural Health* (The National Rural Health Association Supplement), 2003, *19*, 303.
4. According to the Institute for Rural Health Research, the term "Black Belt" has long had a double connotation. The crescent-shaped region known as the Black Belt stretches from across South Texas to Virginia. As noted by Arthur Raper in his 1936 study *Preface to Peasantry,* this region historically has been home to "the richest soil and the poorest people" in the United States.

Booker T. Washington described being asked to define the term "Black Belt." "So far as I can learn," he wrote in his autobiography, *Up from Slavery*, Black Belt "was first used to designate a part of the country which was distinguished by the color of the soil. The part of the country possessing this thick, dark, and naturally rich soil was, of course, the part of the South where the slaves were most profitable, and consequently they were taken there in the largest numbers. Later and especially since the war, the term seems to be used wholly in a political sense—that is, to designate the counties where the black people outnumber the white."

Dr. Washington's analysis still holds true today. Within the roughly two hundred Southern counties that make up the Black Belt, over half the population is African American. In Alabama, it extends from the Mississippi across the heart of the state. Despite rich cultural traditions, the area faces significant socioeconomic problems, including economic stagnation, declining population, low educational attainment, and insufficient health care.

The Robert Wood Johnson Foundation

The Robert Wood Johnson Foundation: 1974–2002

Joel R. Gardner

Editors' Introduction

Although the Robert Wood Johnson Foundation became a national philanthropy only thirty-four years ago, the institution's history and the personalities that have shaped it are important to an understanding of its current philosophy and principles. People often say that a philanthropy can change quickly—especially with the arrival of a new leader. While this has much truth in it, the past does in fact shape thinking and practice at the Robert Wood Johnson Foundation, just as it does in most organizations attempting to play a serious role in American life.

In Volume VIII of the *Anthology*, Joel Gardner, a writer and historian who has conducted oral histories and other historical research on behalf of the Foundation since 1991, and Andrew Harrison, the Foundation's archivist, told the story of the establishment and early years of the Foundation—years in which the Foundation was shaped by the founding chairman of the board, Gustav Lienhard, its first president, David Rogers, and a board that had many personal ties to the founder, Robert Wood Johnson.[1] This chapter by Gardner complements the earlier chapter and takes the Foundation through 2002, when Steven Schroeder retired and Risa Lavizzo-Mourey assumed the role of president and chief executive officer.

While many of the basic approaches to grantmaking that are still evident today—the national program structure, a focus on communications and evaluation, scholarship and fellowship programs, and the testing of new ideas through large demonstration programs—began during the Foundation's first three years, in subsequent years the fruits of these approaches to grantmaking appeared and new approaches were developed to meet changing times and priorities. In this chapter, Gardner weaves the personalities who shaped the Foundation, the impact of their leadership on the Foundation's strategies and programs, and the national environment that influenced the Foundation's grantmaking into a concise history of the Robert Wood Johnson Foundation.

1. Gardner, J. R. and Harrison A. R. "The Robert Wood Johnson Foundation: The Early Years." *To Improve Health and Health Care, Vol. VIII: The Robert Wood Johnson Foundation.* San Francisco: Jossey-Bass, 2005.

—ᴍ—**A** visitor to the Robert Wood Johnson Foundation offices turns off of U.S. 1 in Princeton, New Jersey, onto a curving, country-like road and then into a small, tree-lined parking lot. The Foundation's new building, completed in 2001, rises into an almost bucolic landscape. The front doors lead into a tall atrium. To the left is a large portrait of Robert Wood Johnson himself—the man whose bequest has enabled the Foundation, over its thirty-four year existence, to assume and maintain leadership in the world of health philanthropy. A little beyond is the Foundation's mission statement, a direct descendant of the credo that Johnson developed for his company, Johnson & Johnson.

A photograph on one wall of the long hallway between the entrance and the information center shows David E. Rogers and Gustav O. Lienhard, the president and the chairman, respectively, of the Foundation in its earliest days as a billion-dollar institution. Rogers, the visionary president, looks off into the distance, as though imagining the next program, the next big grant. Lienhard gazes at Rogers, smiling, perhaps knowing that he holds the key to the philanthropic treasury.

Another photograph shows a frame house on Livingston Avenue in New Brunswick, New Jersey—the first home of the Foundation under the leadership of Lienhard and Rogers. The next photos show the first shovelful of earth turned, a cast of board and staff, and the Foundation's trustees, circa 1974, at the site that now houses the Foundation.

—ᴍ— 1972–1976

As the Foundation moved into its new home, it operated within its defined structure and within the goals and guidelines set in 1971 and 1972, the year that the Robert Wood Johnson Foundation became a national philanthropy. The board comprised mostly Johnson & Johnson colleagues and professional acquaintances of Robert Wood Johnson, who had headed the company since 1932. The staff consisted of experienced grant makers and young enthusiasts under the aegis of Rogers, the former dean of the medical faculty at the Johns Hopkins University School of

Medicine and one of the leading figures in American medicine. Lienhard, the chairman, was the linchpin between the board and the staff, the filter through whom ideas were passed to the board.[1]

Lienhard saw himself as both inhibitor and enabler. He held staff members back from proposing grants that he felt the board would not approve, but at the same time, if he believed that an idea was worthwhile, he made every effort to persuade the board to support it. His partnership with Rogers created an equilibrium that enabled the young Foundation and its youthful staff to thrive. For program staff members, the greatest challenge was to create a multi-million-dollar program and design it so that Rogers and then Lienhard would support it.

Three objectives governed the Foundation's early grant making. They were designed to support a system of national health insurance that the Nixon administration and Congress were expected to establish. The three initial objectives were to:

- Expand access to medical care services for underserved Americans (which dominated the Foundation's early grant making).

- Improve the quality of medical care.

- Develop mechanisms for the objective analysis of public policies on health.

To carry out these objectives, the Foundation adopted three approaches: demonstration programs that tested ideas in a number of different locations; training and education of health professionals; and research, evaluation, and policy analysis.

Demonstration Programs

To reach its objective of expanding access to care, the Foundation relied primarily on large demonstration programs to test promising ideas in a number of locations. To administer its early demonstration programs, the Foundation adopted a model by which grants were managed by national program offices, often based in academic medical centers, and counseled by national advisory committees comprised of experts in the field.[2] This model enabled the Foundation to develop demonstration programs that were then evaluated, with the hope that the federal government would respond to successful efforts with additional funding.

The Foundation's first major national demonstration program was the Emergency Medical Services Program. A call for proposals, issued in 1973, described the outcomes the Foundation was seeking, the amounts and the number of the grants that the Foundation would fund, and the criteria that would be applied in the selection of grantees. A grant to the National Academy of Sciences provided support for administration, site visits, and evaluation. This program, which tested different ways of responding to medical emergencies in forty-four different communities, laid the groundwork for the 911 call system that is ubiquitous today.[3] With variations developed over the years, national programs based on the Emergency Medical Services Program model became the norm.

Training and Fellowships

The Clinical Scholars Program provided the template for the second approach—training programs.[4] By selecting sites to provide training and then choosing scholars competitively, the Foundation was able to expand the scope of education in medicine and public health. The Clinical Scholars Program and its early companion, the Health Policy Fellowship Program,[5] provided the model for other scholarship and fellowship programs most recently categorized under the rubric of "human capital." These programs used national program offices to administer them and national advisory committees to select candidates. They provided training to health care professionals, primarily physicians, with the expectation that the graduates would play prominent roles in health policy or academic medicine.

Training and fellowship opportunities were a particularly appropriate way of increasing the number of minority physicians, who were more likely than majority physicians to practice in underserved inner city and rural areas. [6] Scholarships for minority medical students (along with women and medical students from rural areas), a summer enrichment program for minority students in the College of Medicine and Dentistry of New Jersey, and institutional support for Meharry Medical College were among the earliest examples of the Foundation's efforts to address the issue. In the

1980s, the Minority Medical Faculty Development Program (renamed the Harold Amos Medical Faculty Development Program in 2003) and the Minority Medical Education Program (now called the Summer Medical and Dental Education Program) eased the way for more members of racial and ethnic minorities to enter the field of medicine.

The Foundation used a wide range of approaches in carrying out a strong commitment to nursing—a field that Robert Wood Johnson cared deeply about and that he supported in his personal philanthropy. In its efforts to strengthen the nursing profession in the 1970s, the Foundation funded projects in different sites—especially hard-to-reach rural sites—to demonstrate the value of nurse practitioners and physician assistants in providing care to underserved populations. It supplemented demonstration programs with fellowship and scholarship programs, such as the Nurse Faculty Fellowships in Primary Care and the Clinical Nurse Scholars Program.[7] The commitment has continued over the decades with a series of programs to strengthen nursing in hospitals and nursing homes, to improve the quality of home health care and nursing home aides, and to train a corps of leaders of the nursing profession. [8]

Research and Evaluation

That research and evaluation have been an important part of the Foundation's initiatives since the beginning should come as no surprise. Research was essential to the worlds of both Rogers and his closest associate, Robert J. Blendon—one a doctor of medicine, the other of science—and evaluation was important to the board members affiliated with Johnson & Johnson, who were accustomed to carefully evaluated clinical trials.

The demonstration model was most valuable if accompanied by data from the programs and analysis of that data. Moreover, policy was one of the three objectives first set forth by Rogers in the 1972 *Annual Report*, and funding policy implied funding research that could provide the justification for policy recommendations. By farming out evaluations to groups such as the RAND Corporation and Mathematica Policy Research, the Foundation sought to receive unbiased, methodologically sound, and credible reports on the programs it funded. In many ways, the Foundation's strong emphasis on evaluation brought a quantitative imperative that suited both the academics and the businessmen on the board, and broke new ground for foundations.[9]

Today, research and evaluation continue to play a vital role in the Foundation's activities. Members of the research and evaluation staff participate in the development of grants and follow them throughout the process. As initiatives for social change have replaced demonstration projects on the agenda, evaluations now focus less on results and more on learning opportunities.

New Jersey Grant Making

The longest thread in the Foundation's grant making leads back to its commitment to New Jersey. It began in New Brunswick and Middlesex County, the home of Johnson & Johnson. Today the Foundation goes further, with a range of grants across the state, but it has also kept its focus on Robert Wood Johnson's hometown.[10]

It is not surprising that this category has survived; it has always been smaller than the larger objective or goal areas, but always in the balance sheet. After all, the board that led the Foundation in the early 1970s was virtually identical to that which had guided it in Johnson's lifetime, comprising among its ten members five Johnson & Johnson alumni as well as a banker, a doctor, and a judge from the New Brunswick area. The board grew, adding more outside members over the years, but the Johnson & Johnson representation has remained strong, and the commitment to the New Brunswick area unwavering.

New Brunswick grantees that bridge the eras include the Kiddie Keep Well Camp for children with disabilities, the Salvation Army, and the Society of St. Vincent de Paul, but the Foundation also contributed to such urban revitalization projects as New Brunswick Tomorrow. The Foundation's grants helped drive the growth of the Robert Wood Johnson Health Network in New Brunswick, assisted the Center for State Health Policy at Rutgers, and established the New Jersey Health Initiatives Program, now based in Camden, which is a competitive grant program for health and health care organizations within the state.

—ɯɯ— 1976–1986

In 1976, Rogers announced the promotion of Leighton E. Cluff to executive vice president. Cluff, a longtime friend and colleague of Rogers, had joined the Foundation earlier that year as senior vice president to handle management and administration.

As the 1970s progressed, the likelihood of reform in the national health care system diminished, and in 1980 the staff and board revisited the Foundation's objectives. Rogers reported new objectives in that year's *Annual Report.* The first objective addressed access to health care and emphasized programs to expand access for the most underserved groups. The second objective addressed cost and stressed programs to make health care arrangements more effective and care more affordable. The third addressed chronic illness and focused on programs to help people maintain or regain maximum attainable function in their everyday lives.

Of all the concentrations of the Foundation, none has had a longer life, in one variant or another, than access to care. From its earliest days, the Foundation sponsored programs to expand insurance and delivery, to explore prepaid group plans, to promote primary care (or generalist) medicine, and to set up ambulatory care clinics. In the mid-1970s, it supported a program to improve dental care for the handicapped that changed the practice of serving disabled people;[11] primary care training programs for doctors and nurses;[12] regional perinatal service networks that were able to provide better care for premature and low-birthweight infants than individual hospitals could;[13] and a program to improve the practice of medicine in rural areas by developing primary care group practices in remote communities. Rogers wrote in 1978 that the Foundation's grant making was "increasingly directed toward the remaining groups that continue to have problems getting care, especially residents of inner-city and rural areas, children of low-income families, and the low-income elderly."

Between 1982 and 1984, the Foundation began its long commitment to addressing the needs of the chronically ill. The Program for Hospital Initiatives in Long-Term Care (1982–1988) provided funds for hospitals to develop comprehensive initiatives to meet the medical needs of the elderly, and the Rural Hospital Program for Extended-Care Services (1981–1987) established the concept of "swing beds," which could be used for either long-term or short-term patients.[14]

Two programs begun in the 1980s, Health Care for the Homeless and Community Care Funding Partners, broke new ground. In collaboration with the Pew Charitable Trusts, the Foundation developed the Health Care for the Homeless Program (1983–1990), which brought attention to the needs of that underserved, and even ignored, population and served as the model for the Stuart B. McKinney Homeless Assistance Act, the primary federal law providing assistance to homeless people.[15] Under the Community Care Funding Partners Program (1981–1997), the Foundation collaborated with local foundations to support small health centers serving indigent patients. With these two programs, plus a third, the Interfaith Volunteer Caregivers program (1983–1987) that supported interfaith coalitions of congregations whose members volunteered their services to help neighbors in need, the Foundation began to reach out beyond medical centers to a new audience of grantees: community organizations.

In 1983, the Foundation began to seek ways to address the AIDS epidemic.[16] By 1986, two programs were up and running, one through the University of California, San Francisco, that replicated a community-based model of preventing the transmission of HIV and providing supportive services for HIV-positive people, and the other, aimed at children with AIDS, at the Albert Einstein College of Medicine in New York City. The first program, called the AIDS Health Services Program (1986–1992), provided the model for the Ryan White Comprehensive AIDS Resources Emergency Act, the federal law providing funds for AIDS education, prevention, and treatment. Later, Rogers was named vice chairman of the National Commission on AIDS.

From its earliest days, the Foundation committed itself to having a strong communications function. Working with Rogers and Lienhard, Frank Karel, who was named vice president for communications in 1974, essentially created a model of foundation communications. Lienhard, as Karel writes, wanted to "get the word out"—to share information with the field and the public about the programs the Foundation funded and what could be learned from them. But he wanted that word to be about grantees and not the Foundation itself.[17] The Foundation's staff continues to consider clear communications integral to helping its grantees promote better health and health care. Therefore, the Foundation invests substantially in building grantees' capacity to develop communications strategies and in connecting grantees to policy makers and opinion leaders who can help enhance their impact.

Lienhard's health began to decline in 1984, and the board members began a quest for a successor chairman. While their first choice was a retired Johnson & Johnson officer, no one leaped forward to offer his services. In 1985, the board turned to Robert H. Myers, Jr., whose Washington, D.C. law firm had advised the Foundation on legal issues related to the tax code and to the disposition of assets. Though Myers lived in the Washington area, he agreed to spend weekdays in Princeton so that he could oversee the Foundation.

Shortly after Myers's appointment, Waldemar Nielsen's book *The Golden Donors,* the long-awaited follow-up to his first book, *The Big Foundations,* appeared. Since the publication of Nielson's first study of foundations, bequests had added a number of new members to the foundation world. For the Robert Wood Johnson Foundation, Nielsen provided reassurance that its programs and methodology passed his critical tests. He wrote, "In the clarity and ambitiousness of its purposes, in the intellectual power that has governed its strategy and grant making, in the social sensitivity and political skill by which its programs have been shaped, in the able and creative way in which its programs have been managed, and in the general qualities of integrity and independence that have characterized all it has done, the Robert Wood Johnson Foundation is the best of the big foundations today."[18]

In November of 1985, David Rogers had a heart attack. He survived the attack, but, without Lienhard, he no longer had his strongest advocate with the board. In the fall of 1986, only months after *The Golden Donors* had heaped praise on the Foundation, the board provided Rogers a professorship named for his mentor, Walsh McDermott, at Cornell University Medical College and named executive vice president Leighton Cluff as the Foundation's second president.

—ᴍ— **1986–1990**

Lee Cluff first met David Rogers in 1949, when he accepted an internship on the Osler Service at Johns Hopkins Hospital while Rogers was an assistant resident there. Cluff remained at Hopkins, rising through the ranks to become professor of medicine and head of the Division of Allergy and Infectious Disease at the Johns Hopkins University, until 1966, when he moved to the University of Florida as professor of medicine and chairman of the Department of Medicine. During his tenure there, he promoted projects to serve the health and medical needs of the rural communities of central Florida.

Cluff immediately began to place his own presidential imprint on the Foundation. After seeking ideas from leaders in the health field from around the country, he suggested to the board that the Foundation expand the range of its grant making, most notably by focusing even more on community-based organizations. He also recommended that the Foundation support programs aimed at a wider variety of problems, including specific diseases and threats to health.

As a result, the Foundation adopted three broad goals—assisting the most vulnerable individuals, combating specific diseases of regional or national concern, and addressing broad national health issues and concerns—and ten specific priority areas:

1. Infants, children, and adolescents

2. Chronic illness and disability

3. AIDS

4. Destructive behavior, including substance abuse and violence

5. Mental illness, an issue made more difficult by the era's move to deinstitutionalize mental patients

6. Organization and financing of health services

7. Quality of care

8. Ethical issues, including unequal access and the rising field of genetics

9. Health manpower

10. The impact of medical advances

The priorities did not include access. Cluff wrote, "That traditional focus of Foundation support was diminished, in order to direct energies and resources on those populations most likely to be overlooked in a generally improved (albeit still imperfect) health care delivery system."[19]

One of the most important programs to emerge from the Cluff era was SUPPORT, the Study to Understand Prognoses and Preferences for Outcomes and Risks of Treatment, which laid the groundwork for the Foundation's later work with end-of-life issues. The study found that even after intensive training of nurses and physicians who cared for dying patients and counseling for family members, most Americans die in hospitals, often alone and in pain, after days or weeks of futile treatment, with little planning, and at high cost to the institution and the family.[20] Long after Cluff's departure, the Foundation was hard at work to ameliorate the treatment of patients toward the end of their lives.

Cluff paved the way for his successor in other ways. By making substance abuse a priority, he set the stage for the Foundation's later work to combat smoking. And his efforts to engage the issue of AIDS, along with other social and behavioral health problems, presaged the Foundation's later reorganization into health and health care components.

The board had made clear to Cluff that his tenure was to be short. Myers stepped down as chairman of the board in 1988, to be replaced by Sidney F. Wentz, the former chairman and chief executive officer of Crum & Forster, a New Jersey-based insurance holding company. Cluff stepped down in June, 1990, and the board appointed Steven A. Schroeder to succeed him.

—ɯ— 1990–2002

Steven Schroeder brought to the Foundation an orientation and a way of doing business that differed from those of his predecessors. He was a Californian, for one thing, by temperament as well as birth, though edged by more than a decade in the East. A member of the prestigious

Institute of Medicine who had impeccable academic credentials, Schroeder always maintained a commitment to clinical medicine.

Schroeder graduated from Stanford University and Harvard Medical School, then served two years as an epidemic intelligence officer with the Centers for Disease Control and Prevention. After a residency in Boston and various appointments at Harvard, he joined the faculty of the George Washington University Medical Center. He returned to the West Coast as an associate professor in the Department of Medicine at the University of California, San Francisco, where he founded and became chief of the Division of General Internal Medicine.

He arrived at the Foundation in 1990 as its third president, and had an immediate impact. His goal, Schroeder said, was social change, rather than simply grant making.[21] He sought to consolidate the Foundation's program objectives within a limited number of categories in order, as he wrote in the 1990 *Annual Report*, "to help the nation and its health-care system identify and pursue new opportunities to address persistent health problems and to anticipate and respond to significant emerging problems."[22] This led to a restatement of the institution's goals in July of 1990. The new goals were to:

- Assure that Americans of all ages have access to basic health care.

- Improve the way services are organized and provided to people with chronic health problems.

- Promote health and prevent disease by reducing harm caused by substance abuse.

Reining in the cost of medical care, while not a stated goal, remained a principal concern.

Building upon its earlier work in the field, the Foundation began a vigorous campaign to reduce substance abuse, particularly smoking. In the 1992 *Annual Report*, Schroeder listed five main elements in that campaign: establishing substance abuse as the nation's leading health problem; improving prevention and early intervention; reducing demand through community initiatives; reducing harm caused by tobacco; and understanding the causes of substance abuse.

During Schroeder's tenure, the Foundation delivered nearly half a billion dollars in grants to combat tobacco use through policy research, publicity, advocacy, and demonstration programs.[23] The largest program was SmokeLess States, which, under the direction of the American Medical Association, funded state coalitions whose aim was to encourage tobacco control policies, such as prohibiting smoking in restaurants and raising the tax on cigarettes.[24] The Center for Tobacco-Free Kids, established in 1996, was created to serve as a counterbalance to the Tobacco Institute; it played an important and controversial role in the tobacco settlement negotiations.[25] The Foundation also has given continuous support to the public relations campaigns of the Partnership for a Drug-Free America. In addition to its tobacco control programs, the Foundation addressed the problem of youth drinking by establishing programs aimed at curbing alcohol abuse among college students and drinking by high school and even younger students.[26] It also sought to reduce drug abuse through community programs such as Fighting Back and through the advertising campaigns of the Partnership for a Drug-Free America.[27,28]

Twenty years after the Foundation began its grant making based on the assumption that national health insurance was inevitable, the Clinton administration began to address the issue anew. In response, the Foundation undertook four Conversations on Health, in which Schroeder and a group of panelists, usually including Hillary Clinton and Secretary of Health and Human Services Donna Shalala, entertained comments and questions from grass-roots organizations and individuals. The Clinton health care reform initiative failed, and more than ten years later, Conversations on Health and subsequent Foundation-sponsored television programs related to health care reform remain controversial. Schroeder and most health-care professionals saw the activities as nonpartisan—a means of facilitating discussion. Republican politicians and some board members were less impressed, viewing the Foundation's role as having attempted to facilitate the Clinton plan. After that, the Foundation turned to incremental and targeted change.[29]

One of those targets was the coverage of children. In 1997, the Foundation launched the Covering Kids program, at a projected cost of $13 million, to inform low-income families of children in fifteen states that they might be eligible for Medicaid. One month later, Congress passed the $20 billion State Children's Health Insurance Program. The Foundation added $34 million to the pot to help all states let low-income parents know that their children might be eligible for governmental health insurance and to streamline the enrollment process.[30] The program was expanded in 2001 to cover both eligible children and eligible family members.

Building on the SUPPORT research on the care of dying patients, the Foundation developed a comprehensive approach to improving care toward the end of life. It funded, among other things, programs to expand palliative care in hospitals; revise medical and nursing textbooks; commission articles in professional journals; and organize coalitions to improve end-of-life care and encourage people to fill out living wills and other advance directives.[31] It also funded a widely watched documentary by Bill Moyers, *On Our Own Terms,* that provoked a great deal of media attention and public comment.

In the 1990s, the Foundation expanded its Local Initiative Funding Partners Program, which reached out to community philanthropies,[32] and initiated Faith in Action, a program based on the earlier Interfaith Caregivers program, which explored the possibilities of voluntarism through coalitions of faith-based congregations whose members provided services to homebound neighbors.[33]

While the Foundation continued to provide major support to health policy research, perhaps the most important single health policy program to emerge during the Schroeder years was Health Tracking.[34] The immediate impetus was the chaos surrounding the entrance of managed care into the health care marketplace, marked by the dissatisfaction of both physicians and patients. Through a variety of studies, Health Tracking sought to follow and assess the changes wrought by managed care in terms of access, quality, and cost. To carry out Health Tracking, the Foundation established a new organization, the Center for Studying Health System Change, in Washington, D.C. Its reports and publications have contributed to a deeper understanding of the health care landscape, from Capitol Hill to local agencies.

Under Schroeder's twelve-year leadership, the Foundation went through major changes. For one thing, the board of trustees diversified substantially with the inclusion of the first woman, the first African American, and the first person of Latin-American descent. For another, Schroeder redesigned the Foundation so that both health and health care could be addressed equally. Indeed, the transformation of the Foundation into a bicameral institution was the most momentous change in the Foundation's history, in several ways.

First, by making health and health care equivalent, the Foundation departed from its earlier pattern of grant making, which had concentrated largely on health care. Steven Schroeder and former Foundation senior vice president J. Michael McGinnis offered the following comment on the meaning of the change: "for much of its first twenty years the Foundation attended predominantly to the medical care element of its mission . . . By contrast, it neglected the non-medical care factors that influence a person's health, such as choices about smoking, diet, sexual behavior, and physical activity, as well as environmental exposures and other factors—the health dimension of its mission."[35] The shift provided a rationale for funding programs in substance abuse, tobacco, and other social and behavioral areas.

Second, it led to a restructuring of the staff and a reshuffling of personnel. Staff members had to choose whether to concentrate on either health issues or health care issues. The Foundation was reorganized in 1999, with one senior vice president heading the health group and another heading the health care group.

Third, the new structure recognized the Foundation's size, as is appropriate for an institution with $9 billion in assets. With a staff of upward of 200 working in eleven strategic areas, as well as national program directors, the Foundation was a long way from the small, flexible, generalist staff that had marked its earliest days. To fit the growing staff into an appropriate workplace, Schroeder then undertook the expansion of the Foundation's offices, which today dwarf its predecessor (which was incorporated into the new building) in nearly every way.

Schroeder is the first to admit that the changes he wrought were possible only because of the economic boom that accompanied his presidential years. The rising corpus—from $2.9 billion in 1990 to $8.7 billion in 2000—made some sort of restructuring inevitable. Schroeder's first concept—to split the Foundation into four separate, smaller, program-focused foundations—won little support from the board, which preferred to maintain its unified structure. The next idea—health and health care vice presidents under a realigned management structure—was more palatable to the board.

Sidney Wentz retired as board chairman in 1999, and the board appointed Robert E. Campbell, retired vice chairman of the board of directors of Johnson & Johnson, to succeed him. The board also named Schroeder as both president and chief executive officer.

As Schroeder announced his retirement, which took place at the end of 2002, and looked back on his tenure, he shared his thoughts about his successes and failures in the Foundation's *Annual Report* and in a chapter in a book called *Just Money.*[36] Though he was frustrated at the continuing rise in the number of the uninsured and in the failure of the Foundation to effect major changes in coverage, he looked back proudly at its—and his—impact on the fight against smoking, on programs related to end-of-life issues, and on the expansion of coverage of children through state governments.

—⚒— A Conclusion of Sorts

Thanks to a few dedicated men and women, the Robert Wood Johnson Foundation has accepted the challenge of its founder to invest, in effect, in health and health care in the United States. With his colleagues from Johnson & Johnson closely guarding his legacy, and with an energetic and far-seeing staff daring to dream about what might be, the Foundation reached out in ways large and small to reconfigure the landscape.

The largest task—making decent and affordable health care available to all—remains undone. The Foundation's first assumption, that President Richard Nixon would do for national health care what he did with China, turned out to be incorrect. Moreover, its ability to alter the way in which medicine is practiced in the United States was limited by economic and other factors far beyond its control. Hospitals and their staffs grew and shrank. Physicians became generalists, and then they did not. There was a nursing shortage, and then there was not, and then there was again. Managed care seemed so promising, if only doctors and patients would allow themselves to be managed.

But then there are all those programs to serve the underserved in ghettoes and rural areas; AIDS patients and the homeless; children and the elderly. The anti-smoking initiatives have surely saved lives, and end-of-life care is vastly improved.

Seventy years after Robert Wood Johnson set up the Johnson New Brunswick Foundation in order to donate some parkland, he would look on the foundation that bears his name with pride, but also with cognizance of the force that drove him during his lifetime: there is always more to accomplish.

Notes

1. Gardner, J. R. and Harrison, A. R., "The Robert Wood Johnson Foundation: The Early Years." *To Improve Health and Health Care, Vol. VIII: The Robert Wood Johnson Foundation Anthology.* San Francisco: Jossey-Bass, 2005.

2. *See* Hughes, R. G. "National Programs: Understanding the Robert Wood Johnson Foundation's Approach to Grantmaking." *To Improve Health and Health Care, Vol. VIII: The Robert Wood Johnson Foundation Anthology.* San Francisco: Jossey-Bass, 2005.

3. *See* Diehl, D. "The Emergency Medical Services Program." *To Improve Health and Health Care 2000: The Robert Wood Johnson Foundation Anthology.* San Francisco: Jossey-Bass, 1999.

4. Gardner, J., Krevans, J., and Mahoney, M. "A Conversation About the Clinical Scholars Program [with Hal Holman]." *Medical Care,* 2002 (Vol. 40, Supp. 11), 25–31.

   See also Showstack, J., Anderson Rothman, A., Leviton, L. C., and Sandy, L. G. "The Robert Wood Johnson Clinical Scholars Program." *To Improve Health and Health Care, Vol. VII: The Robert Wood Johnson Foundation Anthology.* San Francisco: Jossey-Bass, 2004.

5. *See* Frank, R. "Health Policy Fellowship Program." *To Improve Health and Health Care, Vol. V: The Robert Wood Johnson Foundation Anthology.* San Francisco: Jossey-Bass, 2002.

6. *See* Lowe, J. I. and Pechura, C. M. "The Robert Wood Johnson Foundation's Commitment to Increasing Minorities in the Health Professions." *To Improve Health and Health Care, Vol. VII: The Robert Wood Johnson Foundation Anthology.* San Francisco: Jossey-Bass, 2004.

7. *See* Keenan, T. "Support of Nurse Practitioners and Physician Assistants." *To Improve Health and Health Care 1998–1999: The Robert Wood Johnson Foundation Anthology.* San Francisco: Jossey-Bass, 1998.

8. *See* Newbergh, C. "The Robert Wood Johnson Foundation's Commitment to Nursing." *To Improve Health and Health Care, Vol. VIII: The Robert Wood Johnson Foundation Anthology.* San Francisco: Jossey-Bass, 2005.

9. *See* Knickman, J. R. "Research as a Foundation Strategy." *To Improve Health and Health Care 2000: The Robert Wood Johnson Foundation Anthology.* San Francisco: Jossey-Bass, 1999.

10. *See* Dickson, P. S. "Tending Our Backyard: The Robert Wood Johnson Foundation's Grantmaking in New Jersey." *To Improve Health and Health Care, Vol. V: The Robert Wood Johnson Foundation Anthology.* San Francisco: Jossey-Bass, 2002.

11. *See* Brodeur, P. "Improving Dental Care." *To Improve Health and Health Care 2001: The Robert Wood Johnson Foundation Anthology.* San Francisco: Jossey-Bass, 2001.

12. *See* Isaacs, S. L., Sandy, L. G., and Schroeder, S. A. "Improving the Health Care Workforce: Perspectives from Twenty-Four Years' Experience." *To Improve Health and Health Care 1997: The Robert Wood Johnson Foundation Anthology.* San Francisco: Jossey-Bass, 1997.

13. *See* Holloway, M. Y. "The Regionalized Perinatal Care Program." *To Improve Health and Health Care 2001: The Robert Wood Johnson Foundation Anthology.* San Francisco: Jossey-Bass, 2001.

14. *See* Begley, S. "The Swing Bed Program." *To Improve Health and Health Care, Vol. VI: The Robert Wood Johnson Foundation Anthology.* San Francisco: Jossey-Bass, 2003.

15. *See* Rog, D. J., and Gutman, M. "The Homeless Families Program: A Summary of Key Findings." *To Improve Health and Health Care 1997: The Robert Wood Johnson Foundation Anthology.* San Francisco: Jossey-Bass, 1997.

16. *See* Bronner, E. "Behind the Curve But Leading the Way." *To Improve Health and Health Care, Vol. V: The Robert Wood Johnson Foundation Anthology.* San Francisco: Jossey-Bass, 2002.

17. Karel, F. "'Getting the Word Out': A Foundation Memoir and Personal Journey." *To Improve Health and Health Care 2001: The Robert Wood Johnson Foundation Anthology.* San Francisco: Jossey-Bass, 2001.

18. Nielsen, W. *The Golden Donors.* New Brunswick, N.J. and London: Transaction Publishers, 1985.

19. Cluff, L. E. *Helping Shape the Nation's Health Care System.* Princeton, N.J.: The Robert Wood Johnson Foundation, 1989.

20. *See* Lynn, J. "Unexpected Returns: Insights from SUPPORT." *To Improve Health and Health Care 1997: The Robert Wood Johnson Foundation Anthology.* San Francisco: Jossey-Bass, 1997.

21. *See* Schapiro, R. "A Conversation with Steven Schroeder." *To Improve Health and Health Care, Vol. VI: The Robert Wood Johnson Foundation Anthology.* San Francisco: Jossey-Bass, 2003.

22. Schroeder, S. "President's Message." *Robert Wood Johnson Foundation Annual Report,* 1990.

23. *See* Bornemeier, J. "Taking on Tobacco: The Robert Wood Johnson Foundation's Assault on Smoking." *To Improve Health and Health Care, Vol. VIII: The Robert Wood Johnson Foundation Anthology.* San Francisco: Jossey-Bass, 2005.

24. *See* Gerlach, K. K. and Larkin, M. L. "The SmokeLess States Program." *To Improve Health and Health Care, Vol. VIII: The Robert Wood Johnson Foundation Anthology.* San Francisco: Jossey-Bass, 2005.

25. *See* Diehl, D. "The Center for Tobacco-Free Kids and the Tobacco-Settlement Negotiations." *To Improve Health and Health Care, Vol. VI: The Robert Wood Johnson Foundation Anthology.* San Francisco: Jossey-Bass, 2003.

26. *See* Parker, S. G. "Reducing Youth Drinking: The 'A Matter of Degree' and 'Reducing Underage Drinking Through Coalitions' Programs." *To Improve Health and Health Care, Vol. VIII: The Robert Wood Johnson Foundation Anthology.* San Francisco: Jossey-Bass, 2005.

27. *See* Wielawski, I. M. "The Fighting Back Program." *To Improve Health and Health Care, Vol. VI: The Robert Wood Johnson Foundation Anthology.* San Francisco: Jossey-Bass, 2003.

28. *See* Capoccia, V. A. "The Evolution of the Robert Wood Johnson Foundation's Approach to Alcohol and Drug Addiction." *To Improve Health and Health Care, Vol. IX: The Robert Wood Johnson Foundation Anthology.* San Francisco: Jossey-Bass, 2006.

29. *See* Rosenblatt, R. "The Robert Wood Johnson Foundation's Efforts to Cover the Uninsured." *To Improve Health and Health Care, Vol. IX: The Robert Wood Johnson Foundation Anthology.* San Francisco: Jossey-Bass, 2006.

30. *See* Garland, S. B. "Covering Kids Communications Campaign." *To Improve Health and Health Care, Vol. VI: The Robert Wood Johnson Foundation Anthology.* San Francisco: Jossey-Bass, 2003.

31. *See* Bronner, E. "The Foundation's End-of-Life Programs: Changing the American Way of Death." *To Improve Health and Health Care, Vol. VI: The Robert Wood Johnson Foundation Anthology.* San Francisco: Jossey-Bass, 2003.

32. *See* Wielawski, I. M. "The Local Initiative Funding Partners Program." *To Improve Health and Health Care 2000: The Robert Wood Johnson Foundation Anthology.* San Francisco: Jossey-Bass, 1999.

33. *See* Jellinek, P., Appel T. G., Keenan T. "Faith in Action." *To Improve Health and Health Care 1998-1999: The Robert Wood Johnson Foundation Anthology.* San Francisco: Jossey-Bass, 1998.

34. *See* Newbergh, C. "The Health Tracking Initiative." *To Improve Health and Health Care, Vol. VI: The Robert Wood Johnson Foundation Anthology.* San Francisco: Jossey-Bass, 2003.

35. *See* McGinnis, J. M. and Schroeder, S. A. "Expanding the Focus of the Robert Wood Johnson Foundation: Health as an Equal Partner to Health Care." *To Improve Health and Health Care 2001: The Robert Wood Johnson Foundation Anthology.* San Francisco: Jossey-Bass, 2001.

36. Schroeder, S. A. "When Execution Trumps Strategy," *Just Money: A Critique of Contemporary American Philanthropy.* Karoff, H.P., ed. Boston: The Philanthropic Initiative, 2004.

CHAPTER

10

Engaging Coalitions to Improve Health and Health Care

Laura C. Leviton and Elaine F. Cassidy

Editors' Introduction

For the past twenty years, the Robert Wood Johnson Foundation has funded programs involving state and local coalitions that aim at improving services, advocacy, systems, and changing unhealthy behaviors. These include coalitions to improve tobacco control policies, prevent substance abuse, contain health care costs, expand access to medical care, promote healthy behaviors and lifestyles, expand long-term care options, strengthen mental health services, provide health care services for the homeless, and, most recently, halt the epidemic of childhood obesity and address racial and ethnic disparities in health care.

The Robert Wood Johnson Foundation Anthology has featured a number of chapters that examine the work of coalitions: Irene Wielawski, "The Fighting Back Program," in Volume VII, and "The Free to Grow Program" in Volume IX; Karen Gerlach and Michelle Larkin, "The SmokeLess States Program" in Volume VIII; Susan Parker, "Reducing Youth Drinking: The 'A Matter of Degree' and 'Reducing Underage Drinking through Coalitions'

Programs" in Volume VIII; and Paul Brodeur, "The Injury Free Coalition for Kids" in Volume VII.

In this chapter, Laura Leviton, a senior program officer, and Elaine Cassidy, a program officer, at the Robert Wood Johnson Foundation, examine the Foundation's efforts to build and strengthen community coalitions as a way of bringing about social change. They not only examine what has worked and what has not worked but also explore some central issues, such as the kinds of social change that are suitable for coalitions, the kinds of membership appropriate for coalitions, and the factors that contribute to a coalition's working effectively.

—ɯɯ— **C**oalitions have existed in the United States since the thirteen colonies banded together to share power and address a common problem.[1] Alexis de Tocqueville was the first to note the distinctly American tendency to form associations to deal with specific problems.[2] When a single association cannot solve the problem by itself, it is but a small step to forming a coalition.[3] Over the past forty years, governments and foundations have found it useful to engage state and local coalitions in efforts to improve health and health care. Their approach—including that of the Robert Wood Johnson Foundation—has evolved considerably.

To the best of our knowledge, the first large-scale national initiatives to bring about social change through local coalitions occurred in the 1960s with the initiation of Community Action Programs in the War on Poverty. The Economic Opportunity Act of 1964 required that Community Action Agencies provide for the maximum feasible participation of the poor, members of groups serving the poor, and local public officials. In comparison to the War on Poverty programs, community development programs of the late 1970s and early 1980s put much more power into the hands of government and less in the hands of community coalitions. In the mid-1980s, the federal government and foundations developed a renewed interest in coalitions, particularly comprehensive community coalitions, as a way of bringing about social change.

—ɯɯ— **Comprehensive Community Coalitions**

Beginning in the mid-1980s, the federal Centers for Disease Control and Prevention, the Center for Substance Abuse Prevention, and occasionally the National Institutes of Health began to place coalitions at the center of some of their efforts to promote health and to prevent disease. Two programs from the 1970s had stimulated their interest in a comprehensive approach to community improvement. The North Karelia, Finland, and the Stanford Five-City projects had achieved notable success in modifying risk factors for heart disease by employing comprehensive approaches that included working with schools, businesses, media, churches, and other community institutions to reduce communitywide rates of smoking, lower high blood pressure, and improve diet.[4] The comprehensive, multi-faceted health promotion and disease prevention approach has been an important model ever since for programs ranging from preventing HIV/AIDS and violence to encouraging people to call 911 when they have heart-attack symptoms.[5] In the community development arena, both the federal government and a variety of foundations have turned to coalition models. Congress authorized Empowerment Zones/Enterprise Communities in 1993 and provided flexible grants to promote the revitalization and growth of 105 distressed communities. Along with economic and community development, Congress required broad participation by all sectors of the community.[6]

At roughly the same time, foundations such as Annie E. Casey, Edna McConnell Clark, Ford, John D. and Catherine T. MacArthur, Charles Stewart Mott, Pew Charitable Trusts, and Surdna adopted the approach of Comprehensive Community Initiatives as a way to improve poor urban neighborhoods. Comprehensive Community Initiatives strive to improve distressed neighborhoods through a variety of economic and community development activities. An essential element of this approach is the community coalition that draws together organizations dealing with housing, the local economy, education, health and human services, and other community needs. At the same time, Comprehensive Community Initiatives emphasize participation of the more informal associations and institutions of these neighborhoods' leaders and residents.

In 1990, for example, the Ford Foundation funded the Neighborhood and Family Initiative. Its aim was comprehensive improvement of specific poor neighborhoods in Detroit, Memphis, Hartford, and Milwaukee. Ford awarded grants to the community foundations of these cities to bring together those governmental and non-governmental organizations with power to improve the neighborhoods. The centerpiece of the Neighborhood and Family Initiative was a neighborhood collaborative with the authority to determine what improvements would be made and how they would be made.

Two organizations have provided intellectual leadership to Comprehensive Community Initiatives. The Aspen Institute's Roundtable on Community Change is a forum of experts in the use of community coalitions for social change, and the Chapin Hall Center for Children is a research and development center at the University of Chicago. Both institutions have long argued that a strong theory of change is vital to the work of coalitions, both to guide efforts at comprehensive community improvement and to enable evaluators to reach fair conclusions and draw lessons from the experience.[7] Andrea Anderson, a research associate at the Aspen Roundtable, has written:

> Community initiatives are sometimes planned without an explicit understanding of the early and intermediate steps required for long-term changes to occur; therefore, many assumptions about the change process need to be examined for program planning or evaluation planning to be most effective. A theory of change creates an honest picture of the steps required to reach a goal. It provides an opportunity for stakeholders to assess what they can influence, what impact they can have, and whether it is realistic to expect to reach their goal with the time and resources they have available.

Anderson then goes on to define the theory of change:

> A basic [theory of change] explains how a group of early and intermediate accomplishments sets the stage for producing long-range results. A more complete [theory of change] articulates the assumptions about the process through which change will occur and specifies the ways in which all of the required early and intermediate outcomes related to achieving the desired long-term change will be brought about and documented as they occur.[8]

After evaluating a number of Comprehensive Community Initiatives, the Chapin Hall Center offered some recommendations for philanthropic grant making that could apply to coalitions as well:

- Take extra time to understand communities before making investments.
- Have realistic expectations and align goals accordingly.
- Accept the fact that change is messy, so conflict and risk are inherent to the process.

■ Use a more disciplined process for strategy development, including a better theory of change, better recognition of barriers to change, and an intervention that is of high enough quality, power, pervasiveness, and duration.[9]

—ᗯ— The Evolution of the Robert Wood Johnson Foundation's Work with Community Coalitions

Since 1981, the Foundation has invested $775 million in programs to build and strengthen community coalitions. (For a representative sample, see the appendix.) Among its earliest efforts was Community Programs for Affordable Health Care, which was funded initially in 1981 and continued through 1989.

Community Programs for Affordable Health Care

Co-sponsored by the American Hospital Association and the Blue Cross Blue Shield Association, the purpose of Community Programs for Affordable Health Care was to restrain the rise of health-care costs through broad-based coalitions of health care and other organizations. Intended to be an alternative to the two approaches then being discussed to control costs—government regulation or the wholly voluntary efforts of hospitals and other providers—the program brought together a wide range of stakeholders, such as business, labor, insurers, hospitals, physicians, and consumers, all of whom would work together to keep costs down in their community.

Although the community coalitions were supposed to be the focal point, local control was undermined in two ways. First, the program's national advisory committee was highly prescriptive in its requirements and recommendations. Second, most of the local coalitions did not develop imaginative or aggressive strategies to contain costs. Among other issues the program raised was a tension between top-down leadership and bottom-up control and direction of a program.

The evaluation concluded that the program had produced few measurable effects and presented a variety of reasons that local coalitions were simply not capable of containing costs by themselves.[10] The most important reason was that only the federal government could have achieved a change of the magnitude originally envisioned; local coalitions simply did not have enough clout. The evaluators pointed out that there were probably many health goals that local coalitions *could* achieve, but that they were ill suited as vehicles for containing medical costs. In other words, the premise behind the program—its theory of change—was flawed.

Initiatives of the Late 1980s and 1990s

Despite the failure of Community Programs for Affordable Health Care, the initiative did stimulate greater interest in a coalition approach to the Foundation's work. So did the Comprehensive Community Initiatives approach adopted by other foundations. Several of the large Robert Wood Johnson Foundation initiatives of the late 1980s and the 1990s are similar to the Comprehensive Community Initiative approach. For example, the Urban Health initiative engaged broad community coalitions and stimulated community participation to improve children's health in five American cities. The Free to Grow program supported seventeen Head Start programs by organizing broad-based coalitions to reduce substance abuse in their communities. The Fighting Back program focused on establishing community coalitions composed of local citizens, agencies, and organizations that would work together in combating substance abuse.

As with the Comprehensive Community Initiatives, these programs sometimes experienced struggles for control over the direction of planning and implementation when local coalitions had different expectations from those of program directors.[11] Other Foundation programs also engaged community coalitions, but did not aim for comprehensive change in neighborhoods. For example, the Faith in Action program funded local interfaith coalitions to provide volunteer services such as transportation and household chores to homebound chronically ill people.

In the Fighting Back program, there are echoes of the call for a strong theory of change reminiscent of the Comprehensive Community Initiatives. In brief, the Fighting Back theory of change had two parts:

- Each community had a unique context that affected the nature of its substance-abuse problem. Outside experts would not be familiar with the local context, so effective programs were more likely when local grassroots leadership worked with local health care and social service providers and with the police.

- Existing solutions focused on the reduced availability of drugs, but not on reduced demand. It was assumed that local direction of Fighting Back could reduce the demand for drugs. Citizen participation was needed to change community attitudes and behavior about drug use.[12]

The evaluation of the program concluded that the initiative produced little, if any, change in the use of alcohol and illegal drugs—a conclusion that is vigorously challenged by the program's proponents.[13]

The debate over Fighting Back has been highly revealing about different perspectives on community-based coalitions: on the one hand, some people believe that local coalitions are a way—and perhaps *the* way—to address community health issues. While on the other hand, others doubt that local coalitions can accomplish much of value.[14] These differences of opinion may be easier to resolve than the debaters realize because the theory of change may not have been strong enough for a long enough period of time for the actions of coalitions to be effective. The Fighting Back director, David Rosenbloom, has pointed out that until recently there were no effective strategies—community-based or otherwise—to reduce the demand for harmful substances. Without effective activities to reduce demand, local direction and citizen participation would simply not be sufficient to reduce substance abuse.

For the Foundation, 1996 was a watershed year in thinking about local coalitions, as the Fighting Back program changed both its leadership and its direction.[15] Before 1996, the program was clearly floundering. Coalitions often had cumbersome governance and members had conflicting agendas; proposed activities changed, depending on who showed up at meetings. The new director of Fighting Back guided the remaining coalitions toward more coherent governance and narrower membership, and helped them to focus their program activities. Inclusiveness is an important goal, but at some point there needs to be an agreement to proceed with a plan. Some Fighting Back coalitions were not renewed because they could not change their approach, which discouraged some of their participants from collaborating on projects to address other community problems. The experience has been sobering for Foundation staff members.

~~ Current Foundation Programs

The Robert Wood Johnson Foundation's support of coalition-based programs benefited in many ways from initiatives of the early 1990s. Perhaps the structure and direction of Foundation initiatives have not changed as much as the clarity of expectations from the start of program planning and operation. In the present day, the Foundation strives to convey these expectations in advance. It selects an overall approach, ideally with a strong theory of change, to drive activities. Grantees are expected to adopt the overall direction set forth by the Foundation, but local coalitions have some flexibility to adapt the overall model to their own circumstances. Setting these expectations in advance helps align coalition partners with the Foundation's overall goals and strategies. It also helps avoid some, but not all, struggles for control of the program direction.

Ideally, programs and grantees address a problem for which there are clearly specified activities aimed at solutions. In order for the program to meet its end of this bargain, the theory of change has to be strong or at least plausible, and needs to take into account what is feasible to do in the communities where the coalition operates. With this in mind, the programs rely on local wisdom to make the activities relevant and effective. Two Foundation-funded programs, Allies Against Asthma and Covering Kids & Families, illustrate the diversity of health and health-care problems that are currently being addressed through coalitions.

Allies Against Asthma: A Program to Combine Clinical and Public Health Approaches to Chronic Illness

Of all chronic childhood diseases, asthma is the most common. Although asthma is found in all social classes and racial and ethnic groups, it is most likely to burden children from poor, urban, minority communities. Although significant advances in asthma management have emerged in the past decade, some six million children continue to suffer from the disease. Variations in health-care recommendations and practices, treatment adherence by patients and families, access to high-quality health services, and exposure to high levels of environmental allergens and irritants all undermine the quality of asthma care for many children, especially those from low-income backgrounds. Treatment and prevention can include pressuring landlords to deal with mold and mildew in run-down housing, making sure that the school nurse keeps medication on hand for acute episodes, and helping families understand the ways they can manage their children's illness. Asthma is a complex disease, requiring complex management and the cooperation of many people—circumstances where a local coalition might be able to bring people together who could collaborate in improving care.

In 1998, the Robert Wood Johnson Foundation authorized $12.5 million for the Allies Against Asthma program. The program, which runs over a nine-year period, consists of seven coalition grantees, each comprising stakeholders such as local health-care providers, schools and day care centers, community advocacy groups, businesses, local government organizations, managed care organizations, academic institutions, parent groups, and other community-based organizations. The coalitions' goal is to improve asthma care for children under eighteen years of age, especially those seen under publicly financed systems of care or targeted by safety net providers.

Allies Against Asthma is based on a strong theory of change, both at the level of specific interventions and at the community level. In brief, there is good evidence that asthma interventions are generally effective; what is lacking is a way to get them into widespread use. At the community level, Allies employs the model of comprehensive community-based health promotion, which has often proved more effective than individual, one-on-one patient education. The Allies' theory of change focuses first on developing a manageable and inclusive coalition, which then assesses opportunities for intervention. These interventions are directed toward achieving intermediate results, such as health-provider training or improved management of the disease by the families. The intermediate achievements are expected to affect asthma-related outcomes, including fewer emergency room visits and utilization rates related to asthma. The activities within each of these general components may vary across coalitions, but such variation on the common themes is intentional: the specifics are driven by local context, while the overall model remains the same.

The coalitions have used a variety of strategies to improve pediatric asthma care. Most of the coalitions have educated providers about advances in pediatric asthma treatment and have helped families of children with asthma recognize the conditions that can trigger an attack so as to avoid severe episodes. Allies coalitions also promote policies that help families manage asthma, such as making medication available in schools and child care settings. Coalition members receive training in policy advocacy and support in implementing changes. Like many recent community-based initiatives, Allies seeks a comprehensive change in the way care is delivered, drawing on the cooperation of many organizations and individuals who have the power and resources to make the changes.

Because the activities of the coalitions need to be relevant to the people who are most involved with the problem—parents and children with asthma—the Allies program requires strong community and parental participation in decision making about the activities of the local coalitions. Strong community participation offers opportunities for patients and families to make their voices heard. By inviting community members to participate in early conversations about the Allies coalitions, for example, the program learns about different communities' strengths, needs, and political sensitivities.

The *Alianza Contra el Asma Pediátrica* (Allies Against Pediatric Asthma) in Puerto Rico focuses on the Luis Lloréns Torres public housing project. With over 8,800 residents, it is the largest low-cost housing community in the United States and the Caribbean. About 600 of the project's children have asthma. The *Alianza* uses staff members from both the local public health clinic and the housing project's community center to recruit children with asthma into clinical treatment. In addition to numerous clinic-based, community-based, and school-based activities, the coalition provides information to families about their rights to safe housing for their children, as well as educational sessions and home visits from community health workers.

The *Alianza* directors made a presentation that provided information on the project's strengths, challenges, and achievements.[16] The staff members have long experience with a community-centered approach to public health and health care. They brought key local stakeholders into the coalition. These included AmeriCorps*VISTA volunteers, Líderes Independientes de Luis Lloréns Torres, Luis Lloréns Torres Resident Councils, Head Starts, schools, the apartment complex management corporation, and the police department; islandwide organizations such as APNI (the Association of Parents of Children with Disabilities), ASPIRA (a nonprofit organization devoted to education and leadership development for Puerto Rican youth), Banco Popular of Puerto Rico, Quality for Business Success, the Puerto Rico American Lung Association; and medical-care providers and systems, including the Luis Lloréns Torres Diagnostic and Treatment Center, Medical Card Systems, and the San Jorge Children's Hospital.

There were challenges to the coalition's work. The *Alianza* encountered some clashes within the coalition related to differences in attitudes and values, and also to power and role conflicts among community leaders, other coalition members, and the staff. The directors needed to "balance the community's perceptions of need for services and immediate action with the expectations and requirements of the funding agency and the procedures of the academic grantee institutions," and to "develop trust between the community and university partners," according to the *Alianza* presentation. However, the directors pointed out that these conflicts are a normal part of coalition work. They dealt with them by improving communication, clarifying expectations, using principle-guided conflict resolution, and using language that everyone could understand.

The Allies' evaluation is attempting to determine the effect of the coalitions' work at the individual, community, and population levels. Individual health outcomes for the children and families will be compared with those of similar families living outside the program's geographic areas. These health outcomes include the children's quality of life, daytime and nighttime symptoms, and self-reported hospital and emergency-department visits. Community-level changes include the degree to which asthma action plans are standardized and the growth of policies that promote better asthma care. At a population level, the evaluation is tracking reductions in asthma-related hospitalizations and emergency-department visits.

Because visible changes in population-level health outcomes may not emerge until Robert Wood Johnson Foundation funding of the program has ended, the Allies' evaluation is being conducted in partnership with the federal Centers for Medicare & Medicaid Services and the Agency for Healthcare Research and Quality. They plan to obtain health care utilization data for the Allies' sites and comparison communities for the periods before, during, and after the coalitions' interventions.

Covering Kids & Families

The purpose of Covering Kids & Families is to enroll eligible children and their families in Medicaid and in the State Children's Health Insurance Program, or SCHIP. The original program, Covering Kids, was funded by the Foundation in 1997, and Covering Kids & Families, an extension of the program to involve families as well as their children, was funded in 2001. The program has three goals: outreach to children and families to help them enroll in Medicaid and SCHIP; streamlined state procedures for enrollment and renewal of coverage; and the coordination of benefits across different categories of insurance eligibility. Materials for the program state, "The family should not have to know program details in order to apply for coverage, nor should decisions on coverage be delayed as information is transferred between programs."[17] Funding goes to statewide coalitions, but each state must also have at least two local coalitions. At least half of the funds go to support local coalition activities, which serve as learning laboratories for the statewide coalitions.

In brief, the theory of change behind Covering Kids & Families is as follows: state and local coalitions can overcome specific barriers to enrollment. By getting in touch with families through the institutions they trust (schools, churches, and others), the coalitions can persuade families to enroll. By advocating at the state level for a streamlined enrollment and renewal process, they can overcome bureaucratic barriers to enrollment. By helping to manage the coordination of benefits across different categories of eligibility, the coalitions can prevent the families from being dropped by public insurance. And insurance coverage means that the families' chances to obtain appropriate medical care are greatly increased.

The entire process, however, makes two key assumptions: (1) that the expansion of public insurance eligibility for the poor, seen in the late 1990s, will be maintained; and (2) that publicly insured people will have access to care. The first assumption has been problematic and may have compromised the overall effectiveness of the program. To overcome access barriers, the program's coalitions have undertaken special initiatives to increase access to care.

As of April 2006, 45 state and more than 140 local Covering Kids & Families coalitions were in operation. The coalitions range in size from 5 to 232 members, and membership is fluid and changing.[18] The state coalitions, with a median of 52 members, are generally larger than local coalitions, with a median of 24 members. Most of the coalition membership at both state and local levels comes from community organizations that care for and represent the poor. They bring with them volunteers, credibility, and the trust they have gained in low-income communities. Of the three Covering Kids & Families activities—outreach, simplifying enrollment, and coordinating insurance benefits across programs—the local community organizations clearly have the most resources to bring to bear on outreach. At the state level, they are able to work for their constituencies by advocating streamlined enrollment and preservation of public insurance dollars.

Community-based organizations are a particularly appropriate way to reach rural populations and people facing special cultural and language barriers to public health care coverage.[19] Outreach works through the organizations and community associations upon which these populations depend. These organizations can help overcome mistrust of public agencies, as well as the stigma associated with reliance on public programs. Churches and mosques, for example, can reach out to groups of new immigrants and rural populations. Members of coalitions can also use their knowledge of the community to make their outreach more effective. For example, the Chicago coalition's knowledge of the Korean community led it to advertise the need for enrollment in Medicaid and SCHIP on a Korean-language television soap opera in Chicago.

The state and local coalitions have similar membership, except that there are more government officials in the state coalitions and more school and education representatives in the local coalitions. The involvement of government officials in the state coalitions makes sense since government controls the Medicaid and SCHIP procedures. In the same way, schools are important to local coalitions as places to enroll children, especially during annual back-to-school campaigns.

Relatively few Covering Kids & Families coalition members are individual residents of the affected communities. This offers a distinct contrast to the Allies initiative, in which individual parents participated in the coalitions' decision making. In the context of this program, however, individual community residents bring fewer resources to the table than do the community-based organizations that work on their behalf.

Coalition members provide a variety of resources. In order of frequency, these are: time, help in gaining access to uninsured families and children, help in gaining access to policy makers and influential people, help in mobilizing a constituency in support of Covering Kids & Families goals, access to the media or the public, and funding.

Collaboration often works to overcome conflicting agendas by providing a win-win scenario. The California and New Mexico coalitions, for example, worked with the U.S. Citizenship and Immigration Service (formerly the U.S. Immigration and Naturalization Service) to clarify policy for new immigrants. This collaboration insured that parents received accurate information that their child's enrollment would not jeopardize their own or their child's immigration status. In Las Cruces, New Mexico, the coalition arranged for immigration officials to speak at community meetings about these issues, and handed out materials that spelled out immigrants' rights.[20]

Surprisingly little conflict arose out of the operation of the coalitions. This is probably testimony to the clarity of the goals and process, and the extent to which the state and local partners had accepted them. Conflict is more likely when coalitions are first forming, as the partners test each others' intentions and vie for power and leadership. Conflict is also more likely when goals are unclear, as conflicting agendas can play out. Finally, conflict is more likely when members are in a competition for resources.

Although the theory of change underlying Covering Kids & Families is explicit, coalition members have different priorities, depending on their resources and their roles. Outreach to enroll children and families is the most important goal for local coalition members—understandably, since enrollment is where local coalitions make their biggest contribution. State coalitions report that their most important goals are simplified enrollment and avoiding cutbacks in state funding. The state-level directors generally place coordination of coverage—a very different priority—at the top of their list. They are in a position to see how all the other activities can be defeated—outreach, simplification, and state funding—if there is no coordination. Coalitions can enroll thousands of families, but if they are dropped because of eligibility changes or transitions, the effort is wasted.

According to the evaluation of the program, the coalitions have enrolled thousands of families and children, and they have had some success in streamlining eligibility applications and coordinating benefits. However, tight economic times for states have hindered their efforts. Coalition members mentioned barriers that were beyond their control: state funding issues and new restrictions in Medicaid and SCHIP. The state-level coalitions cited day-to-day obstacles to their work, such as politics, the Medicaid bureaucracy, and a lack of support from state agencies. The evaluation reports noted "a palpable sense of frustration" over these obstacles.[21]

—〰— Concluding Thoughts

Our examination of the Robert Wood Johnson Foundation's strategy in coalition building raises a number of issues concerning coalitions as a vehicle for bringing about social change. Three of them are of primary importance.

Coalitions as an Effective Means for Promoting Social Change

Coalitions have a decidedly mixed record of achievement in reaching their goals. Nationally, some people continue to be profoundly skeptical that local coalitions can achieve very much, and they question whether those coalitions are even appropriate to achieve societal change. Some of this skepticism is based on the mixed track record to date. Some of it is also a reaction to the overuse of coalitions to solve a wide variety of problems. One senior staff member at the Foundation has had a great deal of success in working with coalitions. For that very reason, she understands their limitations. As she pointed out, "We keep pushing coalitions as a way to do our work, but they can be a real waste of time. Why have a coalition when I can identify the right organization that can do the job?" Coalitions take considerable time and energy, so they should never be undertaken lightly. They are not the answer to every social problem.

Finally, some of the skepticism about local coalitions comes from a tendency to "overprofessionalize" the proposed solutions by asserting that the problems of health and health care can be solved only by government and by professionals. The debate about the Fighting Back program illustrates the schism: some say the program has not brought about measurable reductions in substance abuse, and others challenge the methodology or say that it has had positive benefits anyway. The critics doubt that community wisdom and commitment can be sufficient to overcome the overwhelming problems of substance abuse and drug trafficking.

The Need for Strong Theories of Change

The debate over effectiveness misses a central issue: strong theories of change are absolute prerequisites to achieve social change through coalitions. Effective (or at least plausible) interventions are the basis for a strong theory of change: if there is no strong theory, there is no "active ingredient," and therefore no change. Fighting Back illustrates the problem. At the time the program was being developed, no one had any solutions to reducing the demand for drugs—not the community, not the professionals, and certainly not the government. A coalition requires an effective strategy of change to apply to a community problem, just as a hospital needs effective therapy if it is to save lives. Saying that coalitions failed to reduce the demand for drugs is like saying that hospitals fail because people die in them. Both the hospital and the coalition are the vehicles for intervention, not the "active ingredient." Hospitals can be of greater or lesser quality, and local coalitions can operate with greater or lesser direction and force. But these are the vehicles for intervention, not the interventions themselves.

Strong theories of change are important, not just for programs that employ coalitions but for health and social programs of any kind. Theories of change (and a closely related concept, logic models) have long been recognized as essential to assure effective programs and to provide them with a fair and constructive test.[22] In general, evaluators are concerned that the interventions that are tested are simply too puny to make a difference in measurable outcomes.[23]

Interventions need to be of sufficient duration, and be both relevant and powerful enough to produce measurable change. The theory of change highlights these issues for program planners.

We would argue, however, that strong theories of change are especially important in programs that employ coalitions because the coalition members bring a wide variety of other agendas with them. Without a compelling common purpose and way of achieving it—plausible, understandable, and agreed upon by all—coalition members can find it far too easy to capture the effort for their other agendas and divert both resources and activities away from the stated goal. As in the case of certain Fighting Back coalitions, without a central core and agreement to proceed, the agenda and planned activities are vulnerable to constant change.[24]

How to Create and Manage an Effective Coalition Process

Coalitions do not simply appear; they are built. Either they were functioning before a grant was awarded or else the hard work of coalition building has to begin after the award. It is essential to recognize that people build coalitions, not foundations and not their money. Money can assist coalitions, free up resources, and attract attention. Foundations can offer good ideas, skilled facilitators, technical assistance, and networks for sharing. But local leaders build the coalitions. The Foundation's most important error in its early community initiatives was to assume that money would be sufficient to build state and local coalitions. On the contrary, the money can make it seem that there is a coalition when there is none. State and local leaders and organizations come together around Foundation initiatives only when they believe that the purpose of the initiative is consistent with their own common purpose. Foundations engage coalitions; they do not build them.

Community organizers have developed considerable expertise around building and leading coalitions.[25] The Comprehensive Community Initiatives and other recent community-based coalitions highlight the importance of building and leading coalitions correctly. Poorly structured coalitions and poorly understood expectations have derailed community-based efforts. On the other hand, expertise in community organization is seen in the two case studies of Allies Against Asthma and Covering Kids & Families. With a change in leadership, Fighting Back was also able to refocus the remaining coalitions on the work at hand. Considering these and other experiences, we would argue that Foundation-funded coalitions work best when the leadership of a national initiative has expertise in community organization.

There is a range of legitimate models for community coalitions.[26] The degree of shared power with community participants can vary depending on the goal of the coalition. In some cases, all that may be required is community consent or buy-in. The Covering Kids & Families coalitions tended toward this model. In other cases, the program may be committed to solving the problems that the community residents identify, then building capacity and activities to address these problems. The Allies program tended toward this model (with the proviso that activities had to address asthma). The revised Fighting Back program after 1996 was somewhere between the two.

Participation should be dictated by the perspectives and resources that the coalition needs. In the Allies program, the perspective of family members was absolutely critical to ensure the relevance of interventions. In Covering Kids & Families coalitions, direct participation by families was less relevant to the purpose at hand. Other coalition members are usually asked to the table because they have needed resources, or have the know-how for implementation. Resources and know-how are critical, because community-based problem-solving tends to falter at the transition from planning to implementation.[27]

There is a strong tendency for those working with coalitions to conflate the coalition itself with participation by the affected parties. Some funders, and many of those who study coalitions, view the quality and the extent of community participation as an outcome of programs, on a par with program outcomes such as community betterment and health and societal changes. Most of us would agree that community participation is a good thing. If the community is not better off, however, what is the value of the participatory process?

Inclusiveness is not the only criterion for excellence in a coalition. Clarity of purpose and effective governance are at least as important. They are especially important when communities are under stress because of poverty, high crime rates, inequality of resources, or a lack of trust. When the Robert Wood Johnson Foundation invites these community partners to the table, they bring precious commodities: limited time that could be used to solve many other community problems, limited resources that could be applied in many other ways, and personal reputations in the communities where they live. A well-functioning coalition and a clear theory of change can assure that these precious commodities are well-used, and even enhanced.

In sum, debates about the effectiveness of coalitions in health and social programming miss the point: no program can be successful if its theory of change is inarticulate, weak, or built on flawed assumptions. At the same time, as the vehicle of social change, coalitions need good governance, a clear focus, and the right participants at the table. Greater attention to these issues at the planning stage will create a winning proposition for communities and improve the track record for effectiveness of coalition-based programs.

Appendix: Some Major National Programs that Engage Coalitions

Initiative	Dates	Amount
Community Programs for Affordable Health Care	1981–1989	$13,828,000
Community Care Funding Partners Program	1981–1997	$7,151,000
Health Care for the Homeless	1983–1990	$18,082,000
Health Care for the Uninsured	1985–1992	$6,153,000
Fighting Back	1988–2003	$68,365,000
Free to Grow	1992–2006	$13,230,000
Coming Home	1992–2005	$13,004,000
Reducing Underage Drinking Through Coalitions	1995–2005	$19,742,000
Urban Health Initiative	1995–2006	$62,911,000
Covering Kids	1997–2002	$43,930,000
Allies Against Asthma	1998–2006	$12,278,000
Faith in Action	1999–2007	$50,500,000
Covering Kids & Families	2001–2006	$64,863,000

Note: This list is for illustrative purposes and does not include all of the Foundation-funded programs that engage coalitions.

Notes

1. According to the Center for Philanthropy and Nonprofit Leadership, a coalition is "an alliance of individuals and organizations working together on a common purpose." (www.npgoodpractice.org) "Alliances" are relationships of shared power, limited in time and scope. In coalitions, individuals and organizations decide that their own interest is served by ceding some power and resources to a larger alliance. The focus of coalitions that emphasize social change is collaboration, "a process through which parties who see different aspects of a problem can constructively explore their differences and search for solutions that go beyond their own limited vision of what is possible." (Gray, B. *Collaborating: Finding Common Ground for Multiparty Problems.* San Francisco: Jossey-Bass, 1989.)
2. de Tocqueville, A. *Democracy in America: And Two Essays on America.* London: Penguin Classics, 2003.

3. Leviton, L. C., Needleman, C., and Shapiro, M. *Confronting Public Health Risks: A Decision-Maker's Guide.* Thousand Oaks, Calif.: Sage, 1997.

4. Fortmann, S. P., Flora, J. A., Winkleby, M. A., Schooler, C., Taylor, C. B., and Farquhar, J. W. "Community Intervention Trials: Reflections on the Stanford Five-City Project Experience." *American Journal of Epidemiology,* 1995, *142,* 576–586; and Puska, P., Tuomilehto, J., Nissinen, A., Vartiainen, E. *The North Karelia Project—20 Year Results and Experiences.* Helsinki: National Public Health Institute (KTL), 1995.

5. Leviton, L. C. and Guinan, M. E. "HIV Prevention and the Evaluation of Public Health Programs." *Dawning Answers: How the HIV/AIDS Epidemic Has Helped to Strengthen Public Health.* Oxford University Press, Oxford, U.K.: 2002; and Diehl, D. "The Chicago Project for Violence Prevention." *To Improve Health and Health Care, Vol. VIII: The Robert Wood Johnson Foundation Anthology.* San Francisco: Jossey-Bass, 2005; and Luepker, R. V., Raczynski, J. M., Osganian, S., Goldberg, R. J., Finnegan, J. R., Jr., Hedges, J. R., Goff, D. C., Jr., Eisenberg, M. S., Zapka, J. G., Feldman, H. A., Labarthe, D. R., McGovern, P. G., Cornell, C. E., Proschan, M. A., and Simons-Morton D. G. "Effect of a Community Intervention on Patient Delay and Emergency Medical Service Use in Acute Coronary Heart Disease: The Rapid Early Action for Coronary Treatment (REACT) Trial." *Journal of the American Medical Association,* 2000, *284*(1), 60–67.

6. In practice, however, the extent of business and resident participation varied a great deal. See Chaskin, R. J. *Lessons Learned From the Implementation of the Neighborhood and Family Initiative: A Summary of Findings.* Chicago: Chapin Hall Center for Children, 2000.

7. Kubisch, A., Weiss, C. H., Schorr, L. B. and Connell, J. P. *New Approaches to Evaluating Community Initiatives: Concepts, Methods, and Contexts.* Washington, D.C.: Aspen Institute, 1995.

8. Anderson, A. "An Introduction to Theory of Change." *The Evaluation Exchange,* 2005, *XI*(2), 12–19.

9. Brown, P., Chaskin, R., Hamilton, R., and Richman, H. *Toward Greater Effectiveness in Community Change: Challenges and Responses for Philanthropy.* Chicago: Chapin Hall Center for Children, 2003.

10. Brown, L., McLaughlin, C., Cohen, A. B., Cantor, J. C., Schroeder, S. A., Cohodes, D. R., Meyer, J., Stiles, G. M., and Dunlop, J. T. "Constraining Costs at the Community Level: A Critique; Perspectives." *Health Affairs,* 1990, *4,* 5–47.

11. Lindholm, M., Ryan, D., Kadushin, C., Saxe, L., and Brodsky, A. "'Fighting Back' Against Substance Abuse: The Structure and Function of Community Coalitions." *Human Organization,* 2004, *63*(3), 265–276.

12. Saxe, L. and Tighe, E. "The View from Main Street and the View From 40,000 Feet: Can a National Evaluation Understand Local

Communities?" *Evaluation of Health and Human Services Programs in Community Settings: New Directions in Program Evaluation,* Volume 83. San Francisco: Jossey-Bass, 1999.

13. *See* Wielawski, I. M. "The Fighting Back Program." *To Improve Health and Health Care, Vol. VII: The Robert Wood Johnson Foundation Anthology.* San Francisco: Jossey-Bass, 2004.

14. Ibid.

15. Ibid.

16. Lara, M., Pacheco, E., and Rivera, R. *Alianza Contra el Asma Pediátrica en Puerto Rico (Allies Against Asthma in Puerto Rico).* Presentation at the Centers for Disease Control, Atlanta, Georgia, 2002.

17. Southern Institute on Children and Families. *Understanding Policy and Improving Eligibility Systems,* 2002. (http://coveringkidsandfamilies.org/resources/docs/CKFPrimerDec2002.pdf)

18. Lavin, B., Wooldridge, J., Ellis, E., and Stevens, B. *Covering Kids and Families Evaluation: An Analysis of CKF Coalitions Final Report.* Princeton, N.J.: Mathematica Policy Research, Inc., 2004.

19. Howell, E. and Courtot, B. *Covering Kids & Families Evaluation: Targeting Special Populations in the CKF Program: Lessons from Site Visits to Ten States.* Princeton, N.J.: Mathematica Policy Research, Inc., March 29, 2004.

20. Ibid.

21. Hoag, S., Stockdale, H., Courtot, B., Ellis, E., and Gaber, L. *Covering Kids & Families Evaluation: Barriers to Achieving CKF Goals. Highlight Memo No. 10.* Princeton, N.J.: Mathematica Policy Research, Inc., December 22, 2004.

22. Wholey, J. S. *Evaluation: Promise and Performance.* Washington, D.C.: Urban Institute, 1979.

23. Shadish, W. R., Cook, T. D., and Leviton, L. C. *Foundations of Program Evaluation: Theorists and Their Theories.* Newbury Park, Calif.: Sage, 1990.

24. *See* Wielawski, I. M. "The Fighting Back Program." *To Improve Health and Health Care, Vol. VII: The Robert Wood Johnson Foundation Anthology.* San Francisco: Jossey-Bass, 2004.

25. For example: Bracht, N. *Health Promotion at the Community Level: New Advances.* Thousand Oaks, Calif.: Sage, 1990; and Brown, C. *The Art of Coalition Building: A Guide for Community Leaders.* New York: The American Jewish Committee, 1984. Kansas University. "The Community Tool Box." (http://ctb.ku.edu/).

26. Ibid

27. "The Community Tool Box," Centers for Disease Control. PATCH: Planned Approach to Community Health. Atlanta, Ga.: CDC, 1985; and Wandersman, A., and Hallman, W. *Environmental Threats: Perception of Risk, Stress, and Coping.* Presented at the Spanish Congress of Environmental Psychology, Tenerife, Spain, April, 1994.

—ᴡᴡ— Afterword

Shortly after work on this volume of the *Anthology* was completed, Jim Knickman announced that he was leaving the Robert Wood Johnson Foundation to become president and chief executive officer of the New York State Health Foundation, a new philanthropy devoted to improving the health of New Yorkers.

As co-editors of the *Anthology* for the past decade, Jim and I have worked closely on an almost-daily basis. Jim's analytical ability, understanding of health and health care, knowledge of the Robert Wood Johnson Foundation, and high professional standards are unique and have been critical to maintaining the quality and integrity of the *Anthology*. In his new position, Jim will continue to make his mark on health and health care, but he will be sorely missed as co-editor of the *Anthology* series.

S.L.I.

—◊— The Editors

Stephen L. Isaacs, J.D., is a partner in Isaacs/Jellinek, a San Francisco–based consulting firm, and president of Health Policy Associates, Inc. A former professor of public health at Columbia University and founding director of its Development Law and Policy Program, he has written extensively for professional and popular audiences. His book *The Consumer's Legal Guide to Today's Health Care* was reviewed as "the single best guide to the health care system in print today." His articles have been widely syndicated and have appeared in law reviews and health policy journals. He also provides technical assistance internationally on health law, civil society, and social policy. A graduate of Brown University and Columbia Law School, Isaacs served as vice president of International Planned Parenthood's Western Hemisphere Region, practiced health law, and spent four years in Thailand as a program officer for the U.S. Agency for International Development.

James R. Knickman, Ph.D., recently became president and chief executive officer of the New York State Health Foundation, which focuses on improving access to health care and public health and expansion of insurance coverage for New Yorkers. For fourteen years, Knickman was vice president for research and evaluation at the Robert Wood Johnson Foundation where he oversaw a range of grants and national programs supporting research and policy analysis to better understand forces that can improve health status and delivery of health care. In addition, he was in charge of developing formal evaluations of national programs supported by the Foundation and the Foundation's performance assessment system. During the 1999–2000 academic year, he held a Regents' Lectureship at the University of California, Berkeley. Previously, Knickman was on the faculty of the Robert Wagner Graduate School of Public Service at New York University. At NYU, he was the founding director of a university-wide research center focused on urban health care. His publications include research on a range of health care topics, with particular emphasis on issues related to financing and delivering long-term care. He has served on numerous health-related advisory committees at the state and local levels and spent a year working at New York City's Office of Management and Budget. Currently, he chairs the board of trustees of Robert Wood Johnson University Health System in New Brunswick and he is a member of the Board of Directors of the New York Catholic Health Care System. He completed his undergraduate work at Fordham University and received his doctorate in public policy analysis from the University of Pennsylvania.

—⁓— **The Contributors**

Joseph Alper has been a science and health care writer for twenty-six years, and is currently the editor of *Chemistry* magazine and the National Cancer Institute's Nanotechnology in Cancer Website (http://nano.cancer.gov). He has also served as a contributing correspondent for *Science* and as a contributing editor of *Nature Biotechnology* and *Self* magazines. He has also written for a variety of publications, including *Smithsonian, The Atlantic Monthly, Harper's, The New York Times, The Washington Post,* and *Health Magazine,* and has written numerous policy documents for the National Institutes of Health and the National Academy of Science. Alper has won several national writing awards, including the American Chemical Society's Grady/Stack Award for career achievements in science writing and two national writing awards from the American Psychological Association. Alper has also taught journalism and writing at the University of Wisconsin-Madison, Johns Hopkins University, the University of Minnesota, and Colorado State University. He graduated from the University of Illinois-Urbana and received master's of science degrees in biochemistry and agricultural journalism from the University of Wisconsin–Madison.

Paul Brodeur was a staff writer at *The New Yorker* for many years. During that time, he alerted the nation to the public health hazard posed by asbestos, to depletion of the ozone layer by chlorofluorocarbons, and to the harmful effects of microwave radiation and power-frequency electromagnetic fields. His work has been acknowledged with a National Magazine Award and the Journalism Award of the American Association for the Advancement of Science. The United Nations Environment Program has named him to its Global 500 Roll of Honor for outstanding environmental achievements.

Digby Diehl is a writer, literary collaborator, and television, print, and Internet journalist. Recently honored with the Jack Smith Award from the Friends of the Pasadena Public Library, his book credits include *Angel on My Shoulder,* the autobiography of singer Natalie Cole; *The Million Dollar Mermaid,* the autobiography of MGM star Esther Williams; *Tales from the Crypt,* the history of the popular comic book, movie, and television series; and *A Spy for All Seasons,* the autobiography of former CIA officer Duane Clarridge. For eleven years, Diehl was the literary correspondent for ABC-TV's "Good Morning America," and he was recently the book editor for the "Home Page" show on MSNBC. He continues to appear regularly on the morning news on KTLA. Previously the entertainment editor for KCBS television in Los Angeles, he was a writer for the Emmys and for the soap opera "Santa Barbara," book editor of the *Los Angeles Herald Examiner,* editor-in-chief of art book publisher Harry N. Abrams, and the founding book editor of the *Los Angeles Times* Book Review. Diehl holds an M.A. in theatre from UCLA and a B.A. in American studies from Rutgers University, where he was a Henry Rutgers Scholar.

Elaine F. Cassidy, Ph.D., is a program officer in research and evaluation at the Robert Wood Johnson Foundation, where she works on grantmaking related to addiction prevention and treatment, obesity, vulnerable populations, and pioneering ideas. Her work and interests focus primarily on adolescent health and risk behaviors and on school-based interventions, particularly for children and adolescents living in low-income, urban environments. Cassidy is a former school psychologist and trained mental health clinician who has provided therapeutic care to children and families in school, outpatient, and acute partial hospitalization settings. Cassidy holds a B.A. in psychology and liberal studies from the University of Notre Dame, an M.S.Ed. in psychological services from the University of Pennsylvania, and a Ph.D. in school, community, and child-clinical psychology from the University of Pennsylvania.

Joel R. Gardner is a writer and oral historian who specializes in the history of private philanthropy. In that capacity, he has worked as a consultant to the Robert Wood Johnson Foundation since 1991. In addition, he has conducted oral history projects and written histories for The Pew Charitable Trusts and The John D. and Catherine T. MacArthur Foundation. He has written numerous articles for scholarly journals as well as general-interest publications. Most notably, his article "Oral History and Philanthropy: Private Foundations" appeared in the *Journal of American History* in 1992. He has also written histories of Memorial Hospital of Burlington County, New Jersey, and the Tasty Baking Company, and conducted interviews on behalf of the Columbia University Oral History Research Office and the Getty Center for the Arts and Humanities. His interview for Columbia with Charles Scribner, Jr., became *In the Company of Writers,* published in 1991. He holds degrees in French, from Tulane University, and journalism, from UCLA, where he began his oral history career.

Lee Green is an independent writer and journalist. Emphasizing long-form magazine nonfiction and based in Ventura, California, he has pursued stories in Europe, Central America, the Caribbean and throughout the United States. Though he has written for publications as diverse as *The Atlantic, Sports Illustrated,* and *Audubon,* in recent years many of his articles have appeared as cover stories for the *Los Angeles Times Magazine.* Notable among these have been a critique of the U.S. Forest Service, a look at America's secular ethics movement, and an illumination of California's unpreparedness for the state's projected population growth. Green is currently working on a book about U.S. foreign policy.

Risa Lavizzo-Mourey, M.D., M.B.A., is the fourth president and chief executive officer of the Robert Wood Johnson Foundation, a position she assumed in January 2003. Under her leadership, the Foundation implemented a defining framework that focuses its mission to improve the health and health care of all Americans and set bold objectives in nursing, health care disparities, childhood obesity as well as improving public health and quality in the health care system. She originally joined the staff in April 2001 as the senior vice president and director, health care group. Prior to coming to the Foundation, Lavizzo-Mourey was the Sylvan Eisman Professor of Medicine and Health Care Systems at the

University of Pennsylvania, as well as director of the Institute on Aging. Lavizzo-Mourey was the deputy administrator of the Agency for Health Care Policy and Research, now known as the Agency for Health Care Research and Quality. Lavizzo-Mourey is the author of numerous articles and several books, the recipient of many awards and honorary doctorates and frequently appears on national radio and television. A member of the Institute of Medicine of the National Academy of Sciences, she earned her medical degree at Harvard Medical School followed by a masters in business administration at the University of Pennsylvania's Wharton School. After completing a residency in internal medicine at Brigham and Women's Hospital in Boston, Massachusetts, Lavizzo-Mourey was a Robert Wood Johnson Clinical Scholar at the University of Pennsylvania, where she also received her geriatrics training.

Laura C. Leviton, Ph.D., is a senior program officer of the Robert Wood Johnson Foundation. Before joining the Foundation she was a professor of public health at the University of Alabama at Birmingham (UAB) and before that, on faculty of the University of Pittsburgh School of Public Health. Leviton is a leading writer on evaluation methods and practice, in particular for disease prevention. She was president of the American Evaluation Association in the year 2000, coauthored a leading evaluation text, and serves on several editorial boards for evaluation journals. She received the 1993 award from the American Psychological Association for Distinguished Contributions to Psychology in the Public Interest, for her work in HIV prevention and health promotion at the workplace. She served on an Institute of Medicine Committee to evaluate preparedness for terrorist attacks, and was a member of the CDC's National Advisory Committee on HIV and STD Prevention.

David J. Morse is vice president for communications at the Robert Wood Johnson Foundation. From 1997 to 2001, he was director of public affairs for The Pew Charitable Trusts, responsible for managing the Trusts' relationships with media and policymakers and with advising grantees on communications strategies. Before joining Pew, Morse served as associate vice president for policy planning at the University of Pennsylvania, building the university's relations with the federal government, leading efforts to create new mechanisms for financing higher education, and promoting tax policies that preserve incentives for charitable giving. As an aide to U.S. Senators Jacob Javits and Robert Stafford, Morse developed legislation affecting higher education and cultural affairs for the Senate Committee on Labor and Human Resources, and in 1981 directed the President's Task Force on the Arts and the Humanities. He received a B.A. from Hamilton College and an M.A. from The Johns Hopkins University. He serves on the board of the Communications Network and on the Ad Council's Public Policy Advisory Committee, and from 1994 to 2001 taught a public policy course at the University of Pennsylvania's Graduate School of Education.

Mary Nakashian is a consultant specializing in public policy, management, program development and training. She is a former vice president and director of program demonstration at The National Center on Addiction and Substance Abuse (CASA) at Columbia University. For eighteen years, Nakashian worked for state and local governments, including four years as executive deputy commissioner of New York City's Human Resources Administration where she was responsible for the City's welfare, Medicaid, day care, welfare to work and child support enforcement programs. She has written about welfare policy and practice, and writes extensively for the Robert Wood Johnson Foundation. For five years, Nakashian taught at New York University's Robert F. Wagner Graduate School of Public Service.

Carolyn Newbergh is a Northern California writer who has covered health care trends and policy issues for more than twenty years. Her freelance work has appeared in numerous print and online publications. As a reporter for the *Oakland Tribune,* she wrote articles on health care delivery for the poor as well as emergency room violence, AIDS, and the impact of crack cocaine on the children of addicts. She was also an investigative reporter for the *Tribune,* winning prestigious honors for a series on how consultants intentionally cover up earthquake hazards in California.

Irene M. Wielawski is a health care journalist with twenty years experience as a staff writer for daily newspapers, including the *Providence Journal-Bulletin* and the *Los Angeles Times,* where she was a member of the investigations team. She has written extensively on problems of access to care among the poor and uninsured, and other socioeconomic issues in American medicine. From 1994 through 2000, Wielawski—with a research grant from the Robert Wood Johnson Foundation—tracked the experiences of the medically uninsured in twenty-five states following the demise of President Clinton's health reform plan. Other projects in health care journalism since then include helping to develop a pediatric medicine program for public television as well as freelance writing and editing for various publications, including *The New York Times, Los Angeles Times,* and science and policy journals. Wielawski has been a finalist for the Pulitzer Prize for medical reporting, among other solo honors. She is a founder of the Association of Health Care Journalists, and a graduate of Vassar College.

⸺ Index

A

Aaron, Henry, 45
Abney, Kit, 100
Access to Care for the Uninsured collaborative (San Antonio, Texas), 101
Adams, Graham, 176–177, 191, 192
Adams, Kenneth, 88
Aetna, 34, 166
Agency for Health Care Policy and Research, 44
Agency for Healthcare Research and Quality (AHRQ), 44, 73, 233
AIDS Health Services Program, 207
Alabama: medical treatment data for, 35; rural health care programs in, 190
Alabama Department of Community and Rural Medicine, 190
Alabama Department of Public Health, 190
Alabama Power Foundation, 190
Alameda Health Consortium, 85
Albert Einstein College of Medicine, 148, 150, 207
Alderman, Michael, 149, 150, 163, 164, 165, 167*n*.1, *n*.8
Alianza Contra el Asma Pediátrica (Allies Against pediatric Asthma), 231–232
Allies Against Asthma, 229–233, 239, 241
Alper, Joseph, 106, 106*n*.5
American Association of Retired Persons (AARP), 148
American Cancer Society, 148
American Hospital Association, 226
American Lung Association, 148
American Medical Association (AMA), 10, 73
American Public Health Association (APHA), 166–167
AmeriCorps*VISTA, 232

Anderson, A., 242*n*.8
Anderson Rothman, A., 216*n*.4
Annals of Internal Medicine 2003, 38
Annie E. Casey Foundation, 224
Appel, T. G., 219*n*.33
Arkansas, rural health care programs in, 181–185, 192
Arkansas Center for Health Improvement, 181
Arkansas River Valley Rural Health Cooperative, 184
Asbury, C., 106*n*.2
Aspen Institute's Roundtable on Community Change, 224
ASPIRA, 232
Association of American Medical Colleges, 74
Association of Parents of Children with Disabilities (APNI), 232
Austin, Texas, Communities In Charge program in, 85, 97–101

B

Baker, L., 46*n*.7
Balasco, Ernest A., 71
Bamberger, Josh, 142, 143
Banco Popular of Puerto Rico, 232
Bangs, Donald W., 63–64
Baptist Health, 94
Barousky, Marie, 149
Barrand, Nancy, 17, 86, 134, 143
Bassett, W. F., 123*n*.1
Baxter, Ellen, 137
Bayh, Evan, 118
Bayou Teche Community Health Network (ByNet), 186
Beachler, Michael, 171, 172, 173, 174, 175, 176, 177–178, 188, 190, 191, 192–194, 194*n*.3

Begley, S., 217*n*.14

Bella, Melanie, 119, 121

Bellamy, Miles, 90–91

Benjamin, A. E., 22*n*.18, 106*n*.3

Bergeron, Jamie, 192

Berkshire Medical Center, 149, 163

Berkshire Taconic Community Foundation, 149, 150–151, 154, 158

Berkshire Visiting Nurses Association, 147

Berwick, Donald, 42, 55

Big Foundations, The (Nielsen), 208

Bland, Calvin, 6

Blendon, Robert J., 204

Blouin, Richard, 187

Blue Cross Blue Shield, 6, 36, 69, 70, 226

Bornemeier, James, 14, 22*n*.12, 218*n*.23

Bracht, *N.*, 244*n*.26

Braden, Larry, 184

Breakthrough Series programs, 60, 65

Brodeur, Paul, 145, 146*n*.3, *n*.4, 217*n*.11, 222

Brodsky, A., 242*n*.11

Bronner, E., 22*n*.20, 106*n*.1, 217*n*.16, 218*n*.31

Bronner, K. K., 46*n*.7, 47*n*.12

Brook, Robert H., 42, 43, 47*n*.13

Brooklyn Chamber of Commerce, 88, 89–90, 91–92

Brooklyn HealthWorks, 85, 88–93, 103

Broussard, Marcia, 185, 188

Brown, L., 242*n*.10

Brown, Patricia Young, 98, 242*n*.9

Brownlie, Heidi, 70

Bufford, Brenda, 117–118

Bush, George W., 110

Bush, Jeb, 94

ByNet (Bayou Teche Community Health Network), 186

C

California: Communities In Charge program in, 85; health care coalitions in, 235; long-term health care partnerships in, 109–110, 112, 113, 114, 116, 118, 119; medical treatment data for, 35, 36, 39; supportive housing in, 140–142

California HealthCare Foundation, 34

Campbell, Robert E., 215

Cantor, J. C., 104*n*.6, 242*n*.10

Capoccia, V. A., 218*n*.28

CarePartners, 85

Carpenter, Jesse, 129, 130

Carter administration, 82

Cassidy, Elaine, 222

Catline, A., 75*n*.1

Center to Advance Palliative Care, 19

Center for Evaluative Clinical Sciences, 25, 33, 34, 46

Center for Studying Health System Change, 213–214

Center for Substance Abuse Prevention, 223

Center for Tobacco-Free Kids, 212

Centers for Disease Control and Prevention (CDC), 69, 148, 149, 157, 160, 163, 223

Centers for Medicare & Medicaid Services, 73, 115, 233

Chakin, R., 242*n*.9

Chandra, A., 47*n*.11

Chapin Hall Center for Children, 225

Charles Stewart Mott Foundation, 224

Charlotte Hungerford Hospital, 148

Chassin, M. R., 47*n*.13

Children, health care coverage for, 7, 16, 82, 98, 213, 233, 235, 236

Chiles, Lawton, 95

Chronic Care in HMOs program, 56, 59

Chronic care model, 19, 56–58

Chronic Disease Care Program, 54

Chronic illness health care, 49–75; Chronic Care Illness Program and, 58–75; chronic care model of, 19, 56–58; current approaches to, 52–56; RWJF and, 18–19, 54–55

Chronic Mental Illness Program, 54

Clinical Nurse Scholars Program, 204

Clinical Scholars Program, 203

Clinton health care reform effort, 5, 16, 32, 33, 82, 149, 212

Clinton, Hillary Rodham, 16, 212

Clinton, William J. "Bill," 5

Cluff, Leighton E., 206, 208–209, 210, 217*n*.19

Cohen, A. B., 104*n*.6, 242*n*.10

Cohen, Marc, 122
Cohodes, D. R., 242*n*.10
College of Medicine and Dentistry of New
    Jersey, 203
Columbia County Community Healthcare
    Consortium, 158
Columbia County Department of Health,
    158
Coming Home program, 241
Commonwealth Fund, 32
Communities In Charge program, 16,
    79–104; development of, 82–84, 86;
    grantees of, 85; illustrations of, 88–101;
    implementation of, 86–88; review of,
    101–103
Community Care Funding Partners, 207, 241
Community Connecting Program, 182–183
Community Development Financial Institu-
    tions Fund program, 127, 187
Community Health Works, 85
Community Incentive for Diversity project,
    177, 180, 194
Community Match Program, 183
Community Programs for Affordable Health
    Care, 82, 226–227
Community Voices program, 86
Comprehensive Community Initiatives,
    224–225, 227–228, 239
Connecticut: long-term health care partner-
    ships in, 109–110, 112, 114, 115, 116,
    119; medical treatment data for, 29, 31;
    SPARC program in, 147–152, 154–156,
    157–158, 161, 163–167
Connecticut Department of Public Health,
    148, 159
Connell, J. P., 242*n*.7
Conrad *N.* Hilton Foundation, 129
Conversations on Health, 212
Conway, Gordon, 130
Cook, T. D., 243*n*.23
Coordinated Placement program, 189
Cordova, Mark, 64, 65, 66
Cormier, Linda, 147–148, 149, 165–166
Cornell University Medical College, 208
Corporation for Supportive Housing (CSH),
    127, 130, 134, 135–140, 142–144
Cottoms, Naomi, 182–183

Courtot, B., 243*n*.19, *n*.21
Cover the Uninsured Week, 17
Covering Kids & Families, 229, 233–236,
    239, 241
Covering Kids program, 16, 213, 241
Cowan, C., 75*n*.1
Cox, *N.* J., 106*n*.2
Crittenden Community Health Council, 184
Culhane, D. P., 144*n*.3
Culliton, B. J., 75*n*.9
Culp, W. J., 46*n*.5
Cutler, David, 43, 44

D

Dartmouth Atlas of Health Care, 18, 25–47,
    49; practical application of, 42–45;
    RWJF and, 32–34
Dartmouth Medical School, 25
David, Lloyd, 66, 68, 71
De Tocqueville, Alexis, 223, 241*n*.2
Delaney, John, 93
Delta Area Health Education Center, 182
Delta Hills Community Access Program, 184
Dementia Care and Respite Services
    Program, 55
Dental Sealant Days, 99
Dentzer, S., 106*n*.4
Deutsche Bank, 129, 143
DiCamillo, Mark, 10
Dickson, P. S., 217*n*.10
Diehl, Digby, 146*n*.1, *n*.2, *n*.5, 170, 216*n*.3,
    218*n*.25
DiMartino, Donna, 152, 161
Direct Access to Housing program, 142
District of Columbia Primary Care Associa-
    tion, 85
Dougherty, Charles and Gloria, 108
Dunlop, J. T., 242*n*.10
Durenberger, David, 44, 45
Dutchess County, New York Rural Health
    Network, 148
Dyson Foundation, 158

E

East Texas Health Access Network, 189, 190
Economic Opportunity Act of 1964, 223
Edna McConnell Clark Foundation, 224

Effective health care, 38–39

Ellis, E., 243*n*.18, *n*.21

Emergency Medical Services Program, 203

Empowerment Zones/Enterprise Communities, 224

Enterprise Community Partners, 138

Enterprise Corporation of the Delta, 191

Ethnic minorities: health care treatment disparities and, 41; health insurance coverage for, 81; preventive care programs for, 156, 158, 160, 161; preventive health care programs and, 156, 158, 160, 161; at Robert Wood Johnson Foundation, 214, 214; Southern Rural Access Program and, 179, 181, 182–183

F

Fairview Hospital, 163, 166

Faith in Action program, 213, 227, 241

Fannie Mae, 129

Fannie Mae Foundation, 129

Fantel, Donna, 71

Farquhar, J. W., 242*n*.4

Feder, Judy, 120

Federal Rural Health Outreach Grant, 159–160

Felice, John, 136, 137

Fernandopulle, R., 103*n*.3

Fighting Back program, 212, 227–228, 229, 237, 239, 241

Fink, A., 47*n*.13

Fisher, Elliott, 37, 38, 40, 46, 46*n*.1, *n*.6, *n*.7, 47*n*.8, *n*.9, *n*.12

Fleming, David, 156

Fleming, Sandra, 81

Flora, J. A., 242*n*.4

Florida: Communities In Charge program in, 16, 83, 85, 93–96, 101, 102; medical treatment data for, 28, 35, 36

Ford administration, 82

Ford Foundation, 138, 139, 224

Fortmann, S. P., 242*n*.4

Frank, Barney, 131

Frank, R., 216*n*.5

Franklin, W. T., 75*n*.3

Free to Grow program, 227, 241

Freeman, J. L., 46*n*.5

G

Gaber, L., 243*n*.21

Gardner, Joel R., 199, 200, 216*n*.1

Garland, S. B., 218*n*.30

Gaymon, Wilicia, 180

Geisinger Health System, 175

Georgia: Communities In Charge program in, 85; rural health care programs in, 189–190

Georgia Department of Community Health, 189

Gerlach, K. K., 218*n*.24, 221

getCare Health Plan, 85

Gibson, R., 106*n*.5

Gifford, Deirdre, 70, 71

Ginsburg, Paul, 8, 10

Gionfriddo, Paul, 97–98, 101

Gittelsohn, Alan, 28, 29, 46*n*.2, *n*.3, *n*.4

Glenn, William, 179

Golden Donors, The (Nielsen), 208

Golden, Howard, 88

Goldman, Dona, 69, 75*n*.6

Goldman, H. H., 144*n*.4

Gottlieb, D., 46*n*.6, 47*n*.8

Green, Lee, 127–128

Greene, A. Hugh, 94

Greene, John, 113, 118, 122, 123

Griffin, Mark, 178–179

Group Health Cooperative of Puget Sound, 19, 58

Group Health Incorporated (GHI), 90, 91–92

Guinan, M. E., 242*n*.5

Gutman, M., 144*n*.5, 217*n*.15

Guttchen, David, 107, 109, 115, 116, 118, 120, 121

H

Hadley, Jack, 42, 43, 45

Hadley, T., 144*n*.3

Hamilton, R., 242*n*.9

Harold Amos Medical Faculty Development Program, 204

Harrington, Lorie, 149

Harrison, Andrew R., 199, 216*n*.1

Hayes, Katherine, 118, 123

Head Start, 227, 232

Health Access Barriers in the South (HABITS), 186

Health Care Financing Administration, 115

Health Care for the Homeless Program, 54, 133, 134–135, 207, 241

Health care reform: Clinton Administration effort of, 5, 16, 32, 33, 82; historical overview of, 3–22; Robert Wood Johnson Foundation efforts in, 3–22

Health care spending: factors driving, 38–41; geographical variations in, 28–31, 35–37, 39–40

Health Care for the Uninsured Program, 82–83, 241

Health Career Admission Planning Service, 190

Health and Faith Communities Collaborative Project, 181

Health insurance coverage: for children, 7, 16, 82, 98, 213, 233, 235, 236; Communities In Charge program, 79–104; costs of, 8, 11, 13, 107–109; for elders' long-term care, 105–123; expansion of, 15–17; small businesses and, 8, 11, 81, 82–83, 89–92, 94–96, 103; state-level, 107–123

Health Insurance Portability and Accountability Act of 1996, 6

Health Plan Employer Data and Information Set (HEDIS), 39

Health Policy Fellowship Program, 203

Health Resources and Services Administration, 86, 169

Health Tracking, 213

HealthforAll of Western New York, Inc., 85

Healthy Community Access Program, 86, 90, 94, 101

Healthy Futures program, 172, 173

Healthy People 2000 (U.S. Department of Health and Human Services), 153

Heffler, S., 75*n*.1

Heinz, John, 134

Herman, J., 194*n*.3

Hillsborough HealthCare (Florida), 83

Hindmarsh, M., 75*n*.4

Hinds County Health Alliance, 85

Hoag, S., 243*n*.21

Hoffman, Laura, 179

Holloman, Curtis, 191, 194*n*.3

Holloway, M. Y., 217*n*.13

Homebound Adults project, 158

Homeless Families Program, 135

Homeless population: Corporation for Supportive Housing, 135–144; data on, 131–132; RWJF programs and, 129, 133–135; supportive housing for, 127–144

Hospital Corporation of America, 5–6

House Subcommittee on Oversight and Investigation, 156

Housing and Urban Health unit, 142

Howell, E., 243*n*.19

Hudson River Bank & Trust Foundation, 158

Hughes, R. G., 216*n*.2

Human capital, 203

Hurricane Katrina, 10, 100, 170, 171, 188

Hurricane Rita, 170, 171, 188

I

I-Care, 99, 100, 101

Illinois, medical treatment data for, 35

Improving Chronic Illness Care (ICIC), 19, 49, 50, 52, 54, 58–75; components of, 59–60

Indian Health Service, 169

Indiana, long-term health care partnerships in, 109–110, 112, 114, 116, 117, 119

Indigent Care Collaboration (ICC), 85, 97–101

Initiative on Health-Impaired Elderly, 54

Institute for Healthcare Improvement, 18, 19, 59, 60

Institute of Medicine, 9, 10, 19, 41, 49

Interdisciplinary Program of Training, 194

Interfaith Volunteer Caregivers program, 207, 213

Intermountain Healthcare, 44

Isaacs, S. L., 22*n*.11, 217*n*.12

J

Jacksonville, Florida, Communities In Charge program in, 85, 93–96, 102

Jakes, Brian, 186–187, 194

Javits, Carla, 130, 135, 136, 139–140, 142–143
Javits, Jacob, 142
JaxCare, 85, 93–96
Jellinek, P., 219*n*.33
Jessie Ball duPont Fund, 93, 94
John A. Hartford Foundation, 32
John D. and Catherine T. MacArthur Foundation, 224
John, Gregory, 64–66, 74
Johnson & Johnson, 201, 204, 205, 208, 215
Johnson New Brunswick Foundation, 216
Johnson, Robert Wood, 201, 205, 216
Joint Commission on Accreditation of Healthcare Organizations, 59, 73

K

Kadushin, C., 242*n*.11
Kahn, K. L., 47*n*.13
Kansas, Communities In Charge program in, 85
Karel, Frank, 207–208, 217*n*.17
Kaufman, Nancy, 173, 174, 175
Keenan, Terrance, 153, 170*n*.3, 217*n*.7, 219*n*.33
Keesey, J., 47*n*.13
Kennedy, Diane, 180
Kennedy-Kassebaum bill, 6
Kentucky, Communities In Charge program in, 85
Kessler, Mark M., 88, 89, 90, 91–93, 103
Kiddie Keep Well Camp, 205
Kitchen, Ann, 100–101
Knickman, James R., 22*n*.11, 113, 217*n*.9, 245
Kosecoff, J., 47*n*.13
Kubisch, A., 242*n*.7
Kyle, Jonas, 90–91

L

Landis, Ruth, 185
Lara, M., 243*n*.16
Larkin, Michelle L., 218*n*.24, 221
Larson, L., 144*n*.1
Lavin, B., 243*n*.18
Lavizzo-Mourey, Risa, 13, 16, 17, 20, 74–75, 130, 132, 133, 199
Lee, J., 47*n*.11

Leviton, Laura C., 216*n*.4, 222, 242*n*.3, *n*.5, 243*n*.23
Líderes Independientes de Luis Lloréns Torres, 232
Lienhard, Gustav O., 199, 201–202, 207–208
Lindholm, M., 242*n*.11
Lineberry, Isaiah, 175
Local Initiative Funding Partners (LIFP), 146, 152–155, 156, 161, 173, 213
Local Initiatives Support Corporation (LISC), 138
Locum tenens program, 178–179, 193
Long-term care. See Program to Promote Long-Term Care Insurance for the Elderly
Louisiana Public Facilities Authority, 187
Louisiana, rural health care programs in, 185–188
Low Country Health Care Network, 179
Lowe, J. I., 106*n*.6, 216*n*.6
Lucas, F. L., 46*n*.6, 47*n*.8
Luis Lloréns Torres Diagnostic and Treatment Center, 232
Luis Lloréns Torres Resident Councils, 232
Lumpkin, John, 9
Lynn, J., 21*n*.5, 22*n*.21, 218*n*.20

M

MacGregor, A., 194*n*.3
Mack, Mary I., 181
Magan, G. G., 106*n*.6
Magill, Sherry, 94
Mahoney, Kevin, 115–116
Maine: Communities In Charge program in, 85; medical treatment data for, 29
Mangano, Philip F., 131
Marks, James S., 14, 157
Marshall University's Joan C. Edwards School of Medicine, 189
Martin, Amy Brock, 177
Marze, Marsha, 178, 181
Massachusetts: medical treatment data for, 31, 35; Medicare treatment practices in, 29; SPARC program in, 147–152, 154–156, 157–158, 163–167
Massachusetts Department of Public Health, 148, 149
MassPRO, 157

Mathematica Policy Research, 204

Mathews, Craig, 186

McAndrew, Megan, 35, 36

McCall, Nelda, 113, 120

McClellan, M., 47*n*.11

McCulloch, D. K., 75*n*.4

McDermott, Walsh, 208

McGinnis, J. Michael, 214, 219*n*.35

McKay, Hunter, 114

McLaughlin, Catherine, 102, 103, 104*n*.8, 242*n*.10

McVean, John, 136, 137

Meals-on-Wheels, 158

Medicaid: aging population and, 107, 109, 110, 111–116, 118; children's coverage and, 16, 213, 233, 235, 236; Communities In Charge and, 98–99; creation of, 81; financial crisis of, 8, 11, 120; long-term care with, 55, 108, 109, 111–112, 114–115; Partnership for Long-Term Care and, 105–123; rural health care and, 181, 184, 190

Medicaider, 98–99, 101

Medical Card Systems, 232

Medicare: chronic illness and, 55; creation of, 81; geographical spending patterns in, 28–31, 33–42, 44, 45; oversight commission on, 69; prescription drug benefits with, 9, 11; preventive health care and, 157, 163, 165; rural health care and, 181

Medimetrix, 86

Meharry Medical College, 203–204

Meiners, Mark, 111, 114, 118, 119, 120

Melville Charitable Trust, 129

Merrill, Jeffrey, 113

Merritt, N., 47*n*.13

Metraux, S., 144*n*.3

Meyer, J., 242*n*.10

Michael Watson Rural Health Clinic, 179

Michigan, medical treatment data for, 36

Millennial Housing Commission, 131

Milton S. Hershey Medical Center, 175

Minnesota, medical treatment data for, 28, 35

Minority Medical Education Program, 204

Minority Medical Faculty Development Program, 204

Mississippi: Communities In Charge program in, 85; rural health care programs in, 191, 193

Mockenhaupt, R. E., 106*n*.6

Moreno, Paul, 117

Morgante, Sam, 109, 118, 122, 123

Morris, Floyd, 175

Morse, David, 3

Moses, Stephen A., 120, 123*n*.3

Moyers, Bill, 18, 213

Myers, Robert H., Jr., 208, 210

N

Nakashian, Mary, 79, 80

National Academy of Sciences, 203

National Alliance to End Homelessness, 130

National Cancer Institute, 38

National Commission on AIDS, 207

National Committee for Quality Assurance (NCQA), 10, 18, 49, 59, 73

National Health Service Corps, 169

National Immunization Program, 157

National Institute on Aging, 38

National Institutes for Health, 223

National Quality Forum, 18

Needlemann, D., 242*n*.3

Neighborhood and Family Initiative, 224

Neighborhood Health Plan of Rhode Island, 69

Nelson, A. R., 47*n*.10

New Brunswick Tomorrow, 205

New Hampshire, medical treatment data for, 29

New Jersey: medical treatment data for, 35–36, 40; RWJF grant making in, 205

New Jersey Health Initiatives Program, 205

New Mexico: health care coalitions in, 235; medical treatment data for, 35, 39

New Milford Hospital, 148

New York: Communities In Charge program in, 85, 88–93, 103; long-term health care partnerships in, 109–110, 112, 114, 116, 117, 119; medical treatment data for, 35, 36; SPARC program in, 147–152, 154–156, 157–158, 160, 163–167; supportive housing in, 136–138

New York State Department of Health, 148

New York Times, 71, 149, 164

Newbergh, Carolyn, 25, 217*n*.8, 219*n*.34

Nichols, Kristy, 186

Nielsen, Waldemar, 208, 217*n*.18

Nixon administration, 82, 202, 215

Nordstrom, Nikki, 67–68, 74

North Carolina, Indigent Care Collaboration in, 99

North Karelia, Finland project, 223

Northern Berkshire County Committee, 152

Northern Dutchess Hospital, 148

Nurse Faculty Fellowships in Primary Care, 204

O

Obesity, RWJF and, 9–10, 12, 14–15

Office of Rural Health, 176–177, 178, 180–181

O'Kane, Margaret, 45

Older adults. See Program to Promote Long-Term Care Insurance for the Elderly

Olson, Mary, 182

Omnibus Budget Reconciliation Act of 1993 (OBRA 1993), 118–119

On Our Own Terms (Moyers), 18

Oregon, Communities In Charge program in, 85

Orleans, Tracy, 59

Orr, Robert, 118

Osborne, Henry, 95

P

Pacheco, E., 243*n*.16

Palm Beach County Community Health Alliance, 101

Park, R. E., 47*n*.13

Parker, Susan G., 218*n*.26, 221

Parks, Jim, 187

Partnership for a Drug-Free America, 212

Partnership to End Long Term Homelessness, 129–131

Partnership for Long-Term Care. See Program to Promote Long-Term Care Insurance for the Elderly

Pathman, Don, 193

Patient Outcomes Research Teams, 44

Patrick and Catherine Weldon Donaghue Medical Research Foundation, 152

Pechura, C. M., 216–217*n*.6

Penn State College of Medicine, 175

Pertschuk, Michael, 14

Pew Charitable Trusts, 127, 133, 137, 138, 139, 207, 224

Pfizer Foundation, 158

P4P project, 73

Philanthropic Collaborative for a Healthy Georgia, 189

Pillow, Gil, 183

Pillow, John, 183, 184

Pinder, E. L., 46*n*.6, 47*n*.8

Piney Woods Area Health Education Center, 189, 190

Pittsfield Board of Health, 149

Poirier, Rhonda Davis, 93, 94, 95, 96

Polyclinic, 61, 63–68, 74

Practice Management Technical Assistance program, 189

Practice Sights program, 169–170, 172–173

Preference-sensitive health care, 39–40

Prescription for Life initiative, 160

Prevention Sundays, 158

Preventive health care, 12–15. See also Sickness Prevention Achieved Through Regional Collaboration

Price, M. J., 75*n*.4

Program on Chronic Mental Illness, 134

Program for Hospital Initiatives in Long-Term Care, 206

Program to Promote Long-Term Care Insurance for the Elderly, 105–123; assessment of, 120–123; obstacles toward implementation of, 118–120; regulatory problems and, 115–118

Project Access, 85, 99, 101

Project H.E.R.O.A., 149

Project Open Hand, 141

Project Stay Put, 180

Puerto Rico, *Alianza Contra el Asma Pediátrica* in, 231–232

Puerto Rico American Lung Association, 232

Q

Quality for Business Success, 232

Quality Partners, 69

R

Rance, Rosalie, 89

RAND Corporation, 204

Reach Out program, 170

Redford, M. Robert, 184–185

Reducing Underage Drinking Through
Coalitions, 241

Reifler, B. V., 106*n*.2

Republicans, national health care coverage
and, 212

Resnik, Diana, 97

Rhode Island: Improving Chronic Illness
Care program in, 51–52, 68–71; medical
treatment data for, 29

Richman, H., 242*n*.9

Rivera, R., 243*n*.16

Robert Wood Johnson Foundation (RWJF):
chronic illness and, 13, 49–75; Communities In Charge program and, 79–104;
demonstration programs of, 202–203;
health care coalitions and, 221–244;
healthy lifestyle encouragement by, 13–
15; historical overview of, 5–22, 199–215;
homeless services programs, 127–144;
impact framework strategy by, 4; Johns
Hopkins University and, 201–202, 209;
Johnson & Johnson and, 201, 204, 205,
208, 215; and New Brunswick, New
Jersey, 201, 205; New Jersey grant making
efforts and, 205; 1986–1990 activities
of, 209–210; 1990–1992 activities of,
210–215; 1976–1986 activities of,
206–208; 1972–1976 activities, 201–205;
Partnership for Long-Term Care and,
105–123; and preventive health care,
12–15, 145–167; quality of health care
and, 13, 18–19, 37–38; research and
evaluation by, 204–205; rural health care
and, 148, 159–160, 169–195; training
fellowships and, 203–204

Robert Wood Johnson Foundation (RWJF)
Annual Report (1972), 204

Robert Wood Johnson Foundation (RWJF)
Annual Report (1980), 206

Robert Wood Johnson Foundation (RWJF)
Annual Report (1990), 211

Robert Wood Johnson Foundation (RWJF)
Annual Report (1992), 211–212

Robert Wood Johnson Foundation (RWJF)
Annual Report (2002), 215

Robert Wood Johnson Health Network, 205

Rockefeller Foundation, 129, 130

Rog, D. J., 144*n*.5, 217*n*.15

Rogers, David E., 199, 201–202, 204, 206,
207, 208, 209

Rosenblatt, Robert, 22*n*.15, 79, 104*n*.7,
218*n*.29

Rosenbloom, David, 228

Ross, Carolee, 51–52

Ruddock, Joyce, 107, 121

Rural Business Enterprise, 177

**Rural health care programs, 169–195;
SPARC project and, 159–160. See also
Southern Rural Access Program**

Rural Health Outreach, 148

Rural Health Policy Office (U.S. Health
Resources and Services Administration),
148, 159

Rural Health Revolving Loan Program, 177

Rural Hospital Program for Extended-Care
Services, 207

Rural Medicaid Scholars program, 190

Rush, Colette, 65, 66

Rutgers Center for State Health Policy at
Rutgers—the State University, 205

Ryan, D., 242*n*.11

Ryan White Comprehensive AIDS Resources
Emergency Act, 207

S

St. Christopher's Hospital for Children
(Philadelphia), 6

St. Francis Hospital (Dutchess County, New
York), 149

St. Francis residence facilities (New York
City), 137

St. Vincent's Hospital (New York City), 137

Salvation Army, 205

San Antonio, Texas, Communities In Charge
program in, 101

San Francisco Department of Public Health,
142

San Jorge Children's Hospital, 232

Sandorf, Julie, 136–138, 142–144

Sandy, Lewis G., 32–33, 216*n*.4, 217*n*.12

Saxe, L., 242*n*.11, 243*n*.12

Schapiro, R., 218*n*.21

SCHIP (State Children's Health Insurance Program), 7, 16, 82, 98, 213, 233, 235, 236

Schooler, C., 242*n*.4

Schorr, L. B., 242*n*.7

Schroeder, Steven A., 12, 32, 33, 104*n*.6, 172, 174, 175, 199, 210–215, 217*n*.12, 218*n*.22, 219*n*.35, *n*.36, 242*n*.10

Schultz, Pat, 62

Schwarting, Cathy, 179, 180

Science journal, 28

Section 8 housing vouchers, 134

Shadish, W. R., 243*n*.23

Shalala, Donna, 212

Shapiro, M., 242*n*.3

Sharon Hospital, 148, 152–153, 161, 163

Sharp, S. M., 46*n*.7, 47*n*.12

Shelton, Steven R., 191

Shenson, Douglas, 146, 149, 150, 151–152, 153–154, 157, 164–165, 167*n*.1, *n*.7

Shepherd, Joyce, 184

Showstack, J., 216*n*.4

Shuffield, Paul, 182

Sickness Prevention Achieved Through Regional Collaboration (SPARC), 145–167; Federal Rural Health Outreach Grant and, 159–160; future of, 163–166; origins and early activities of, 149–152; Robert Wood Johnson Foundation and, 152–156; Vote and Vaccinate Project of, 161–163

Skinner, Jonathan S., 38, 40, 41, 46, 46*n*.1, 47*n*.9, *n*.11, *n*.12

Small business health insurance, 8, 11, 81, 82–83, 89–92, 94–96, 103

Smedley, B. D., 47*n*.10

Smile Alabama!, 190

Smith, C., 75*n*.1

SmokeLess States program, 212

Smyth, Henry R., 106*n*.2

Snyder, R. E., 22*n*.18, 106*n*.3

Society of St. Vincent de Paul, 205

Solis, Jeanne, 185–186

Solomon, D., 47*n*.13

Somers, Stephen, 110–111, 115, 133–134, 143

Song, P., 104*n*.8

South Carolina Medical Association, 180

South Carolina, rural health care programs in, 176–181, 191, 193, 194

South Carolina Rural Interdisciplinary Program of Training (SCRIPT), 177, 180

Southeast Louisiana Area Health Education Center, 186

Southern Bancorp, 182

Southern Financial Partners, 182

Southern Regional Health Consortium, 191

Southern Rural Access Program, 169–195; in Arkansas, 181–185; leadership and, 190; loan funding and, 191–192; in Louisiana, 185–188; origins of, 172–176; recruitment and retention, 188–189; rural health networks, 189–190; in South Carolina, 176–181

Southwest Louisiana Area Health Education Center, 185–186

Special Committee on Aging, 157

Staiger, D., 47*n*.11

Stanford Five-City project, 223

Staresnick, Michael, 109, 121

Starr, S. S., 103*n*.3

State Children's Health Insurance Program (SCHIP), 7, 16, 82, 98, 213, 233, 235, 236

Stevens, B., 243*n*.18

Stewart B. McKinney Act, 133

Stewart, Kate, 192

Stiles, G. M., 242*n*.10

Stith, A. Y., 47*n*.10

Stockdale, H., 243*n*.21

Stoller, Terry, 87, 92, 102

Stringfellow, Arnold, 140–142

Stuart B. McKinney Homeless Assistance Act, 207

Stucker, Virgil, 150, 151, 152

Study to Understand Prognoses and Preferences for Outcomes and Risks of Treatment (SUPPORT), 18, 210, 213

Stukel, T. A., 46*n*.6, 47*n*.8, *n*.12

Summer Medical and Dental Education Program, 204

Supply-sensitive health care, 40–41

Supportive housing, 127–144

Supportive Services Program in Senior Housing, 54
Surdna Foundation, 224
Susan B. Anthony Award for Excellence in Research on Older Women and Public Health (Aetna), 166–167

T

Takada, Adrianna, 112, 122
Taking Health Care Home, 139
Taylor, C. B., 242*n*.4
Taylor, E. F., 104*n*.8
Texas: Communities In Charge program in, 85, 97–101, 102; medical treatment data for, 35; rural health care programs in, 189, 190, 191
Tighe, E., 243*n*.12
To Err is Human 1999 (Institute of Medicine), 10
Tobacco, programs to control, 7, 13–15
Trail, Mervin, 185
Travis County Communities In Charge project, 97–101, 102
Tri County Rural Health Network (Arkansas), 182, 183
Tri-County Health Care Safety Net Enterprise (Oregon), 85
Tronolone, Michael, 61, 67
Tuskegee Area Health Education Center, 190
21st Century Challenge Fund, 171, 173, 181, 189, 190

U

Unequal Treatment: Confronting the Racial and Ethnic Disparities in Health Care (Institute of Medicine), 41
Uninsured Americans: local efforts to cover, 79–104; number of, 81; RWJF efforts to cover, 15–17. See also Health insurance coverage
United Health, 34
United Healthcare, 69, 70–71
U.S. Congress: children's health care coverage and, 213; community development and, 224; homelessness and, 131, 133; long-term care and, 110; Medicaid program and, 110, 115–116, 118–119, 122–123; medical spending and, 45, 73, 115; national health care coverage and, 6, 7, 81–82, 202
U.S. Department of Agriculture, 176, 177, 187
U.S. Department of Housing and Urban Development (HUD), 127, 134, 135
U.S. Department of the Treasury, 127, 187
U.S. Government Accountability Office, 157
U.S. Health Resources and Services Administration, 59, 148, 159, 189
U.S. News & World Report, 41
University of Alabama Medical School (Tuscaloosa), 190
University of California, San Francisco, 207
University of Chicago, 225
University of Pennsylvania, 132, 133
University of South Carolina, 177
Urban Health initiative, 227, 241
Urbina, I., 75*n*.8
Utah, medical treatment data for, 40

V

Vassar Brothers Hospital, 149
Vermont, medical treatment data for, 28–29
Visiting Nurse Services of Connecticut, 148
Vote and Vax Project, 146, 161–163, 167
Vuris, Mildred, 98

W

W. K. Kellogg Foundation, 86
Wachovia Corporation, 178
Wagner, Edward, 49–50, 56, 57, 58, 59, 61, 72, 75*n*.4
Walton Family Foundation, 182
War on Poverty, 223
Warren, A., 104*n*.8
Warren, D., 194*n*.2
Washington (state), Improving Chronic Illness Care program in, 61–68, 74
Washington, D.C.: Communities In Charge program in, 85; homelessness in, 129
Washington State Collaborative, 65
Weicker, Lowell, 116
Weiner, Joshua, 121, 122, 123*n*.6
Weiss, Anne, 55, 88, 102, 103, 191, 194

Weiss, C. H., 242*n*.7

WellPoint, 34

Wennberg, John E., 25, 26, 27, 28–31, 32–34, 36, 37, 38, 40, 42, 43, 44, 45, 46, 46*n*.1, *n*.2, *n*.3, *n*.5, *n*.6, *n*.7, *n*.8, *n*.9, *n*.12, 55

Wentz, Sidney F., 210, 215

Wessel, D., 47*n*.14

West Virginia, rural health care programs in, 191

West Virginia Department of Health & Human Resources, 188–189

West Virginia Rural Health Infrastructure Loan Fund, 191

West Virginia University, 188–189

West Virginia's Recruitable Community project, 188–189

Whang, Judith, 82, 83

Wholey, J. S., 243*n*.22

Wielawski, Irene M., 25, 49, 50, 146*n*.6, 170*n*.1, *n*.2, 194*n*.3, 218*n*.27, 219*n*.32, 221, 243*n*.13, *n*.24

Wilkins, Mitch, 178

Willis, Floyd, 96

Windleby, M. A., 242*n*.4

Winslow, C. M., 47*n*.13

Wood River Health Services, 51–52, 62, 71

Wooldridge, J., 243*n*.18

Y

Yale-Griffin Prevention Research Center, 156–157, 158

Z

Zerhouni, Elias, 73–74

—w—Table of Contents

To Improve Health and Health Care 1997

Foreword
Steven A. Schroeder

Introduction
Stephen L. Isaacs and James R. Knickman

Acknowledgments

1 **Reach Out: Physicians' Initiative to Expand Care to Underserved Americans**
Irene M. Wielawski

2 **Improving the Health Care Workforce: Perspectives from Twenty-Four Years' Experience**
Stephen L. Isaacs, Lewis G. Sandy, and Steven A. Schroeder

3 **A Review of the National Access-to-Care Surveys**
Marc L. Berk and Claudia L. Schur

4 **Expertise Meets Politics: Efforts to Work with States**
Beth A. Stevens and Lawrence D. Brown

5 **The Media and Change in Health Systems**
Marc S. Kaplan and Mark A. Goldberg

6 **Addressing the Problem of Medical Malpractice**
Joel C. Cantor, Robert A. Berenson, Julia S. Howard, and Walter Wadlington

7 **Unmet Need in the Community: The Springfield Study**
Susan M. Allen and Vincent Mor

8 **Unexpected Returns: Insights from SUPPORT**
Joanne Lynn

9 **Developing Child Immunization Registries: The All Kids Count Program**
Gordon H. DeFriese, Kathleen M. Faherty, Victoria A. Freeman, Priscilla A. Guild, Delores A. Musselman, William C. Watson, Jr., and Kristin Nicholson Saarlas

10 **The Homeless Families Program: A Summary of Key Findings**
Debra J. Rog and Marjorie Gutman

11 **The National Health and Social Life Survey: Public Health Findings and Their Implications**
Robert T. Michael

–ᴠᴠ–Table of Contents
To Improve Health and Health Care 1998–1999

Foreword
Steven A. Schroeder

Introduction
Stephen L. Isaacs and James R. Knickman

Acknowledgments

Combating Substance Abuse

1 **Adopting the Substance Abuse Goal: A Story of Philanthropic Decision Making**
Robert G. Hughes

2 **Tobacco Policy Research**
Marjorie A. Gutman, David G. Altman, and Robert L. Rabin

3 **The National Spit Tobacco Education Program**
Leonard Koppett

4 **Alcohol and Work: Results from a Corporate Drinking Study**
Thomas W. Mangione, Jonathan Howland, and Marianne Lee

Increasing Access to Care

5 **Influencing Academic Health Centers: The Robert Wood Johnson Foundation Experience**
Lewis G. Sandy and Richard Reynolds

6 **The Strengthening Hospital Nursing Program**
Thomas G. Rundall, David B. Starkweather, and Barbara Norrish

Improving Chronic Care

7 **Faith in Action**
Paul Jellinek, Terri Gibbs Appel, and Terrance Keenan

8 **Providing Care—Not Cure—for Patients with Chronic Conditions**
Lisa Lopez

9 **The Mental Health Services Program for Youth**
Leonard Saxe and Theodore P. Cross

Communications

10 **The Foundation's Radio and Television Grants, 1987–1997**
Victoria D. Weisfeld

A Look Back

11 **Support of Nurse Practitioners and Physician Assistants**
Terrance Keenan

–ᴍᴍ–Table of Contents

To Improve Health and Health Care 2000

Foreword
Steven A. Schroeder

Introduction
Stephen L. Isaacs and James R. Knickman

Acknowledgments

Access to Care

1 **School-Based Health Clinics**
Paul Brodeur

2 **Expanding Health Insurance for Children**
Marguerite Y. Holloway

3 **The Minority Medical Education Program**
Lois Bergeisen and Joel C. Cantor

Services for People with Chronic Conditions

4 **Coming Home: Affordable Assisted Living for the Rural Elderly**
Joseph Alper

5 **Adult Day Centers**
Rona Smyth Henry, Nancy J. Cox, Burton V. Reifler, and Carolyn Asbury

6 **The Program on Chronic Mental Illness**
Howard H. Goldman

Research

7 **Research as a Foundation Strategy**
James R. Knickman

8 **Linking Biomedical and Behavioral Research
for Tobacco Use Prevention: Sundance and Beyond**
Nancy J. Kaufman and Karyn L. Feiden

Collaboration with Other Philanthropies

9 **The Local Initiative Funding Partners Program**
Irene M. Wielawski

A Look Back

10 **The Emergency Medical Services Program**
Digby Diehl

Appendix

Twenty-Five Years of Emergency Medical Systems: A Retrospective
James C. Butler and Susan G. Fowler

—ᵐᵐ—Table of Contents

To Improve Health and Health Care 2001

Foreword
Steven A. Schroeder

Editors' Introduction: Grantmaking Insights from The Robert Wood Johnson Foundation *Anthology*
Stephen L. Isaacs and James R. Knickman

Acknowledgments

Inside the Foundation

1 Expanding the Focus of The Robert Wood Johnson Foundation: Health as an Equal Partner to Health Care
J. Michael McGinnis and Steven A. Schroeder

2 "Getting the Word Out": A Foundation Memoir and Personal Journey
Frank Karel

Programs

3 Children's Health Initiatives
Sharon Begley and Ruby P. Hearn

4 The Changing Approach to Managed Care77
Janet Firshein and Lewis G. Sandy

5 Integrating Acute and Long-Term Care for the Elderly
Joseph Alper and Rosemary Gibson

6 The Workers' Compensation Health Initiative: At the Convergence of Work and Health
Allard E. Dembe and Jay S. Himmelstein

7 Sound Partners for Community Health
Digby Diehl

A Look Back

8 The Regionalized Perinatal Care Program
Marguerite Y. Holloway

9 Improving Dental Care
Paul Brodeur

Collaboration with Other Philanthropies

10 Partnership Among National Foundations: Between Rhetoric and Reality
Stephen L. Isaacs and John H. Rodgers

—ɯ—Table of Contents

To Improve Health and Health Care Volume V

Foreword
Steven A. Schroeder

Editors' Introduction: Strategies for Improving Access to Health Care—Observations from The Robert Wood Johnson Foundation *Anthology* Series
Stephen L. Isaacs and James R. Knickman

Acknowledgments

Programs

1 **The Nurse Home Visitation Program**
   Joseph Alper

2 **Tuberculosis: Old Disease, New Challenge**
   Carolyn Newbergh

3 **Programs to Improve the Health of Native Americans**
   Paul Brodeur

4 **Service Credit Banking**
   Susan Dentzer

5 **Consumer Choice in Long-term Care**
   A. E. Benjamin and Rani E. Snyder

6 **The Health Policy Fellowships Program**
   Richard S. Frank

A Closer Look

7 **Recovery High School**
   Digby Diehl

8 ***On Doctoring*: The Making of an Anthology of Literature and Medicine**
   Richard C. Reynolds and John Stone

A Look Back

9 **The Foundation and AIDS: Behind the Curve but Leading the Way**
   Ethan Bronner

Inside the Foundation

10 **Program-Related Investments**
   Marco Navarro and Peter Goodwin

11 **Tending Our Backyard: The Robert Wood Johnson Foundation's Grantmaking in New Jersey**
   Pamela S. Dickson

–ᴍ–Table of Contents
To Improve Health and Health Care Volume VI

Foreword
Steven A. Schroeder

Editors' Introduction
Stephen L. Isaacs and James R. Knickman

Acknowledgments

Section One: Reflections on Health, Philanthropy, and The Robert Wood Johnson Foundation

1 A Conversation with Steven A. Schroeder
Renie Schapiro

Section Two: Improving Health Care

2 The Health Tracking Initiative
Carolyn Newbergh

3 Practice Sights: State Primary Care Development Strategies
Irene M. Wielawski

4 The Foundation's End-of-Life Programs: Changing the American Way of Death
Ethan Bronner

Section Three: Improving Health

5 The Center for Tobacco-Free Kids and the Tobacco-Settlement Negotiations
Digby Diehl

6 Helping Addicted Smokers Quit: The Foundation's Tobacco-Cessation Programs
C. Tracy Orleans and Joseph Alper

7 Combating Alcohol Abuse in Northwestern New Mexico: Gallup's Fighting Back and Healthy Nations Programs
Paul Brodeur

Section Four: Strengthening Human Capacity

8 Building Health Policy Research Capacity in the Social Sciences
David C. Colby

9 The Robert Wood Johnson Community Health Leadership Program
Paul Mantell

Section Five: Communications

10 The Covering Kids Communications Campaign
Susan B. Garland

Section Six: A Look Back

11 The Swing-Bed Program
Sharon Begley

~ɯ~ Table of Contents

To Improve Health and Health Care Volume VII

Foreword
Risa Lavizzo-Mourey

Editors' Introduction: Observations on Grantmaking from The Robert Wood Johnson Foundation *Anthology* Series
Stephen L. Isaacs and James R. Knickman

Acknowledgments

Section One: Targeted Portfolio

1 **The Fighting Back Program**
Irene M. Wielawski

2 **Join Together and CADCA: Backing Up the Front Line**
Paul Jellinek and Renie Schapiro

3 **The Robert Wood Johnson Foundation's Efforts to Contain Health Care Costs**
Carolyn Newbergh

4 **The Teaching Nursing Home Program**
Ethan Bronner

Section Two: Human Capital Portfolio

5 **The Robert Wood Johnson Clinical Scholars Program**
Jonathan Showstack, Arlyss Anderson Rothman, Laura C. Leviton, and Lewis G. Sandy

6 **The Robert Wood Johnson Foundation's Commitment to Increasing Minorities in the Health Professions**
Jane Isaacs Lowe and Constance M. Pechura

7 **The National Health Policy Forum**
Richard S. Frank

Section Three: Vulnerable Populations Portfolio

8 **The Injury Free Coalition for Kids**
Paul Brodeur

9 **The Homeless Prenatal Program**
Digby Diehl

Section Four: Pioneering Portfolio

10 **The Robert Wood Johnson Foundation's Response to Emergencies: September 11th, Bioterrorism, and Natural Disasters**
Stephen L. Isaacs

–ᴡ–Table of Contents

To Improve Health and Health Care Volume VIII

Foreword
Risa Lavizzo-Mourey

Editors' Introduction
Stephen L. Isaacs and James R. Knickman

Acknowledgments

The Editors

The Contributors

Section One: National Programs

1 **Taking on Tobacco: The Robert Wood Johnson Foundation's Assault on Smoking**
James Bornemeier

2 **The SmokeLess States Program**
Karen K. Gerlach and Michelle A. Larkin

3 **Reducing Youth Drinking: The "A Matter of Degree" and "Reducing Underage Drinking Through Coalitions" Programs**
Susan G. Parker

4 **The Robert Wood Johnson Foundation's Commitment to Nursing3**
Carolyn Newbergh

5 **The Turning Point Initiative**
Paul Brodeur

Section Two: A Closer Look

6 **The Chicago Project for Violence Prevention**
Digby Diehl

Section Three: Inside The Robert Wood Johnson Foundation

7 **The Robert Wood Johnson Foundation: The Early Years**
Joel R. Gardner and Andrew R. Harrison

8 **National Programs: Understanding The Robert Wood Johnson Foundation's Approach to Grantmaking**
Robert G. Hughes

–ɯ–Table of Contents
To Improve Health and Health Care Volume IX

Foreword
Risa Lavizzo-Mourey
Editors' Introduction: Still Swinging for the Philanthropic Fences?
Stephen L. Isaacs and James R. Knickman
Acknowledgments

Section One: From the Foundation's Vulnerable Populations Portfolio

1 Free to Grow
Irene M. Wielawski

2 Improving Health in an Aging Society
*Robin E. Mokenhaupt, Jane Isaacs Lowe,
and Geralyn Graf Magan*

Section Two: From the Foundation's Targeted Portfolio

3 The Robert Wood Johnson Foundation's
Efforts to Cover the Uninsured
Robert Rosenblatt

4 The Robert Wood Johnson Foundation's Safety Net Programs
James Bornemeier

5 The Medicaid Managed Care Program
Marsha R. Gold, Justin S. White, and Erin Fries Taylor

6 The Evolution of the Robert Wood Johnson Foundation's
Approach to Alcohol and Drug Addiction
Victor A. Capoccia

Section Three: A Closer Look

7 Students Run LA
Paul Brodeur

Section Four: Pro le

8 Terrance Keenan: An Appreciation
Digby Diehl

Section Five: Issues in Philanthropy

9 Public Scrutiny of Foundations and Charities:
The Robert Wood Johnson Foundation's Response
Susan Krutt and David Morse